When the impossible becomes possible

The path to self-mastery and letting go

Author

Laurent Zecchinon

Title

When the impossible becomes possible - the path to self-mastery and letting go
First edition.

ISBN : 9798870088266

Illustration and photo: Aimy Zecchinon

Website

https://laurentzecchinon.com

Facebook Page (in French)

https://www.facebook.com/lzecchinon.coaching.biohacking

YouTube Channel (in French)

Laurent Zecchinon - Coaching & Biohacking

https://www.youtube.com/channel/UCFZc-S7wxQgUMG_EufSIz6w

Linkedin Profile

https://www.linkedin.com/in/laurent-zecchinon/

DEDICATION

"The biggest plight of the human race is knowing you have more potential, but not utilizing it." Dale Carnegie

This book is dedicated to you, dear reader, who has chosen to be better today than you were yesterday.

If, in addition, you are a parent or grandparent, my dearest wish is that it will help you to better accompany the younger generations.

May the path of self-mastery and letting go take you where you have never gone before.

DISCLAIMER

TABLE OF CONTENTS

ACKNOWLEDGEMENTS

"If I have seen further than others, it is by standing upon the shoulders of giants." Sir Isaac Newton

Thank you to all the people who have contributed, directly or indirectly, to the writing of this book.

Between the various coaches and authors listed in the "References" section and the many trainers I have had the pleasure and privilege of working with in different fields, the list is long. But I would like to mention Tony Robbins in particular, who is a huge source of inspiration for me.

I have a special thought for the people, family, and friends, who have accompanied me on this path of self-mastery and letting go, sometimes for decades. They will all recognize themselves (which, by the way, ensures that I don't forget anyone).

1 - INTRODUCTION

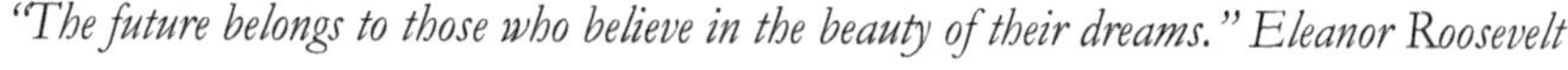

"The future belongs to those who believe in the beauty of their dreams." Eleanor Roosevelt

"If you want something you've never had, you have to do something you've never done."
Thomas Jefferson

"What we can or cannot do, what we consider possible or impossible, is rarely a function of our true capability. It is more likely a function of our beliefs about who we are."
Tony Robbins

"The only limit to your success is your imagination and commitment." Tony Robbins

WHEN THE IMPOSSIBLE BECOMES POSSIBLE

"The only impossible journey is the one you never begin." Tony Robbins

Making the impossible possible sometimes comes down to very small things, usually repeated with regularity.

The most important of these is certainly your definition of the impossible, and the subjective element that comes into play, based on your current knowledge, past experiences, and beliefs. Change these and you will change your definition of the impossible; it is as simple as that.

Take **Siri Lindley**, for example. In the early 90s, she decided to become Triathlon World Champion... even though she could barely swim. By dint of hard work and the implementation of intelligent strategies, she succeeded some ten years later, in 2001. She also won the 2001 and 2002 ITU Triathlon World Cup series. But her story doesn't end there. In 2019, she was diagnosed with acute myeloid leukemia with less than 5% chance of survival. She told herself she was more than a statistic and chose to act, once again putting the necessary strategies in place. The following year, the results of her last bone marrow biopsy were unequivocal: she was cured! A miracle? Perhaps... But what if it was due to the repetition of different habits, the ones that make the difference between success and failure?

THE PATH TO SELF-MASTERY AND LETTING GO

"The ultimate aim of karate lies not in victory or defeat, but in the perfection of the character of its participants." Gichin Funakoshi

Ever since I was a child, I have had a passion for martial arts, and notably for karate, which I have now been practicing for over 35 years (with periods of interruption). In particular, I appreciate the notion of the **path**, the idea that the most important thing is to progress day by day through regular practice (we will see in chapter 4 that there is a particular way to practice effectively).

In Taoism, we also find the notions of Yin and Yang, symbolized by the circle on the cover of this book, which illustrate the complementary nature of opposites, one not existing without the other. Yin is presented by the dark areas and Yang by the light areas. In this way, I am convinced that the path to making the impossible possible involves both self-mastery and letting go.

Self-mastery allows us to give the best of ourselves in order to realize our wildest dreams, and to inspire those around us to do the same.

Letting go is about believing in the magic of something greater than ourselves, whether you call it the Universe, the Quantum Field, God, Allah, or whatever name is most appropriate for you.

It is indeed important to remember that what we want for ourselves is not necessarily the best thing for the whole.

ACHIEVE EXTRAORDINARY RESULTS

"The difference between ordinary and extraordinary is that little extra." Jimmy Johnson

The results you achieve depend on 3 things that influence each other:

- how you feel (your **energy**),
- how you think (your **mindset**) and
- how you act (your **performance**).

In an environment that challenges and supports you, you can thrive and develop if you have the tools you need to face the challenges.

Conversely, an environment that demands a lot of you without providing you with the physical, mental, and spiritual skills you need to meet these challenges can be toxic.

Toxic environments are characterized by unhealthy competition, mockery of those who are different or who don't measure up to the norm, little attention to well-being and, ultimately, isolation, stress and burn-out.

This book aims to bring together a wealth of information, principles, strategies, and tools that, when applied regularly and wisely, will enable you to make the impossible possible.

That is the best I can wish for you.

2 - MASTER YOUR ENERGY

"The number one key to success in life is to master your own state. If you can manage and master your states, there is nothing you can't do." Tony Robbins

"Human beings are designed to be strong, happy and healthy." Wim Hof

"Energy and persistence conquer all things." Benjamin Franklin

The way you feel will have a major influence on the results you achieve. When you feel good and full of energy, you will have better ideas and more motivation to act and give your best.

In fact, we should speak of energy in the plural. In their book "The Power of Full Engagement", **James Loehr** and **Tony Schwartz** identify 4 types of energy:

- physical energy,
- emotional energy,
- mental energy and
- spiritual energy.

I would add two other energies:

- sexual energy, with its masculine and feminine components, which we all possess, whatever our gender or sexual orientation. We are back to Yin and Yang... and
- quantum energy, more subtle but nonetheless vital.

Let's take a closer look.

PHYSICAL ENERGY

"No work is stressful. it is your inability to manage your body, mind and emotions that make it stressful." Sadhguru

Physical energy broadly defines the **quantity** of energy you have available (high or low). It depends mainly on the following factors:

-   your circadian rhythm (sleep and light),
-   the foods and beverages you consume,
-   how you move and breathe, and
-   your ability to detoxify.

Biohacking

In this field, I have become a great believer in Biohacking, a non-dogmatic approach combining ancestral knowledge with the latest scientific discoveries. One of its basic principles is to think in terms of signals and effects.

For example, exposing yourself to natural light from the moment you wake up will enable you to synchronize your circadian (day-night) rhythm and produce the right hormones at the right time, so that you are energized during the day and ready to rest at night. If, on the other hand, you expose yourself to blue light from screens in the evening, you will receive an energizing signal when you are supposed to be in recovery mode at that time of day.

The biohacker's priority is to use natural, free resources first (e.g. exposing yourself to natural light by going outdoors). When this is not possible, use alternatives such as blue-light-blocking glasses if you have to work or consult screens at the end of the day.

Biohacking is a true philosophy that enables you to live a healthy, fulfilled, and successful life, beyond the limiting and even erroneous dogmas that our society promotes today.

The tree of diseases

"A healthy man wants a thousand things, a sick man wants only one."
Confucius

Most of today's illnesses, such as diabetes, asthma, cardiovascular disease, arthritis, obesity, autoimmune diseases, neurodegenerative diseases, anxiety, depression, and various forms of cancer, have **more in common** than we think.

Inspired by the model of **Frank Lipman**, a functional physician, and taken up by **Ronan Diego de Oliveira** in the Mindvalley Holobody certification program I took a few years ago, these diseases can be likened to the foliage of a tree.

The trunk would represent all the processes leading up to it, such as **inflammation**, oxidative stress and hormonal, neurotransmitter, mitochondrial, immune, digestive, detoxifying, and musculoskeletal imbalances.

The roots represent the common causes of **lifestyle imbalances**, including nutrition, recovery, beliefs, physical activity, environmental exposure (light, toxins, and microbes), medications, relationships and genetics. The latter explains why the same imbalances (which can also add up to cause more deleterious effects) will lead to different illnesses depending on the individual.

As our society is currently unfortunately more oriented towards a system of diseases (junk food and pollution → diseases → pill medicine), the latter being very lucrative, than towards a system of health (prevention such as we find more in the East), it is up to you to make your choice, and decide whether or not to prioritize your lifestyle to live better, more fulfilled and more successful... keeping in mind your responsibility towards your children and the following generations.

Self-mastery also, if not primarily, involves acquiring more **critical thinking** skills by asking yourself the right questions. You are the CEO of your health and your life. Not a pharmaceutical company for whom illness is a lucrative business. I would like to make it clear that I am not against all drugs or all pharmaceutical companies. I am against unjustified excess.

Sleep and recovery

Good sleeping conditions can be summed up as follows: total darkness, temperature close to 18°C, between 6 and 8h30 of sleep starting no later than 11pm, at least 2h between the last meal and bedtime, and if possible 2h of abstinence from artificial blue light before bedtime. Also remember to sleep a multiple of 90 minutes (roughly corresponding to the length of a sleep cycle), to avoid waking up half-asleep.

For faster sleep, fewer night-time awakenings and a better quality of time spent sleeping, try a weighted blanket. Sleeping with a (light) weight on your body, relaxes the nervous system (like when you're hugged or kissed), leading to an increase in serotonin and melatonin while reducing cortisol levels in the body. In short, everything you need for a good night's sleep. It would even seem that weighted blankets are particularly useful for children with autism or Asperger's syndrome.

In 2018, I had the privilege of taking part in a **Wim Hof** seminar outside Amsterdam. Nicknamed "The Iceman", he has some twenty Guinness Book World Records to his credit, including:

- running a half-marathon above the Arctic Circle, barefoot and in shorts,
- swimming 66 meters under the ice,
- hanging by one finger at an altitude of 2000 meters,
- climbing Kilimanjaro in shorts,
- running a half-marathon in the Namibian desert without drinking water,
- staying in an ice barrel for over 112 minutes.

While intensive training has taught him to control his breathing, heart rate and blood circulation, and to withstand extreme temperatures, Wim is convinced that we are all capable of such feats. His method is based on three fundamental pillars: **breathing** (hyperventilation and retention), progressive **exposure to the cold** and **mental focus** (aided by the other two). He teaches it all over the world, not only to celebrities, professional athletes, Navy Seals etc., but to everyone.

His method also boasts exceptional results in the **health** field, validated by scientific research. In an experiment carried out in 2014, practitioners of his method were able to control their sympathetic nervous system and immune response after injection of a bacterial endotoxin. Indeed, they showed lower fever symptoms, lower levels of pro-inflammatory mediators, and higher levels of plasma adrenaline, compared to the control group who had not been trained in the method. Incredibly, the training of the first group lasted only 10 days. These data (and more to come) are reinventing our understanding of the human body and opening up tremendous prospects in the management of many contemporary diseases whose common thread is inflammation.

Heat exposure, for example in a sauna for fifteen to thirty minutes, also generates numerous benefits. A study of over 2,000 Finns showed that those who took the sauna between 4 and 7 times a week were 50% less likely to die of cardiovascular disease, and 40% less likely to die of premature death (compared to those who went to the sauna only one day a week).

Regular sauna use can also help you to

- detoxify your body of heavy metals, chemicals, and toxins,
- increase the resistance of your cells through the production of heat shock proteins,
- significantly improve your heart health through the production of red blood cells and the reduction of CRP, a biomarker of inflammation,
- boost the strength of your immune system and
- improve your deep sleep cycles.

In addition to the effects of natural versus artificial light mentioned above, you can also increase your physical contact with the Earth ("**earthing**" or "grounding"). Do you remember the last time you walked barefoot, and the beneficial effect it had on you? We now know that this contact allows you to pick up negative ions (which is not the case when you walk in shoes with insulating soles), resulting in the following effects:

- a powerful antioxidant effect through the neutralization of free radicals,
- reduced inflammation and pain,

- reduced stress,
- stimulation of the immune system,
- a beneficial effect on the cardiovascular system,
- better sleep,
- better recovery from jet lag,
- slower aging and
- protection against the harmful influence of electromagnetic fields.

Here too, Biohacking can help you if you can't go barefoot: there are very affordable mats and even bed sheets that can be plugged into an earth socket to provide the same effects. This will be more beneficial if you spend a lot of time behind a computer, which by its very nature generates electric and electromagnetic fields that induce **nervous fatigue**. For a more in-depth look at the subject, I refer you to the video I made on the subject (in French) with my friend Hugues Ostoja-Kuczynski, geobiological engineer (https://youtube.com/live/8k7ZSoVnyBM?feature=share).

Don't hesitate to call on his geobiological services if you suspect your home is having a negative effect on your sleep and energy. You may be surprised by the impact of your environment, and in particular the presence of watercourses or GSM antennas in your neighborhood.

Finally, we are not all the same when it comes to circadian rhythms. There are in fact 4 forms of the gene regulating our interaction with and dependence on it. The 4 resulting chronotypes are personified by animals whose distribution in the population and optimal rising and setting times are as follows:

- the bear (around 55% of the population): 7am-11pm,
- the lion (around 15-20% of the population): 5am-9pm,
- the wolf (approx. 15-20% of the population): 9am-midnight and
- the dolphin (around 10% of the population): 6am-11pm (with fragmented sleep).

Your performance will therefore vary according to your **chronotype**, meaning that the times of day when you perform best may be different from one person to another.

What is more, your chronotype can influence your life as a couple. For example, if a lion and a wolf are a couple, they will need to avoid having important discussions when they're getting up or going to bed, because if one of them is in full possession of his or her means (the one who initiates the discussion in general), there will always be one who is half asleep, which obviously won't encourage a quality exchange and may even create unnecessary tension. So remember to adapt your pace of life and work to your chronotype as much as you can; it will be all the better for your health, your performance and your zest for life.

Nutrition

"Let food be thy medicine and medicine be thy food." Hippocrates

Nutrition is probably the sector where the mass of contradictory information is the most overabundant, not only because of the financial potential linked to weight loss, but also because **personalization** is an essential factor. We don't all have the same needs and constraints. For example, a food that is excellent for you may be toxic for me, or vice versa.

To get straight to the point, eating correctly can be summed up as follows:

- consume the macro- (proteins, fats, and carbohydrates) and micronutrients (vitamins and minerals) you need to develop, function and regenerate optimally, in sufficient quantities and without excess,
- avoid toxic compounds (added sugars, processed fats, preservatives, allergens) as much as possible.

In other words:

- less industrial, more homemade food (with more "real" organic),
- less sugar, more fruit, and vegetables,
- less bad fats and more good fats,
- less soda and alcohol, more water.

Based on my personal experience, I have often found in my coaching sessions a deficit in proteins, vitamins, and minerals, as well as an excess of calories and processed foods.

Another important aspect will be to limit the period of time during which you eat to 8 to 12 hours a day (to allow the body to recover and "cleanse" itself). It's also possible to add periods of complete fasting if you are so inclined.

In Okinawa, a Japanese island in the East China Sea that is part of the **Blue Zones** (those regions of the world where the longevity of the inhabitants is well above average), it is customary to fill the stomach only to around 80%. This avoids overloading the digestive system while maintaining a more reasonable caloric intake. Give it a try and you'll feel the benefits! As much as I love sharing a good meal in a restaurant with good company, I often think that it makes me eat more than I should, and more than my body needs. Occasionally, this is of course of no great consequence (and can even help to make up for certain deficiencies), but if repeated too regularly...

When you eat is also important. Remember, I mentioned above the circadian rhythm, our internal 24-hour clock; our bodies have different needs at the beginning and end of the day and produce different hormones accordingly. As a general rule, opt for richer meals at the beginning and middle of the day, and lighten them in the evening (unless you need to recover more after a day's effort, for example during a sporting competition). It is also advisable to eat proteins and fats in the morning, and proteins with carbohydrates for a snack around 4PM. In the first case, as well as increasing satiety, lipids promote the transport of tyrosine, an amino acid involved in the synthesis of dopamine, a neuromediator responsible for alertness and motivation. In the second, carbohydrates promote the transport of tryptophan, an amino acid involved in the synthesis of serotonin, which regulates mood, stress, sleep, and appetite. As you can see, we need more dopamine at the start of the day, and more serotonin in the evening.

Recently, I was talking to a friend who confided in me that she was having problems concentrating on her goals, and sometimes even **procrastinating**. It quickly became apparent that she had two bad habits with detrimental consequences on her dopamine production: the first was that she started her day by listening to podcasts on her smartphone (wearing out her dopamine by giving her the illusion of reward), the second was that she ate breakfast with sugary cookies (preventing her from producing enough). Remember, your **lifestyle** is the cause or solution to many of your problems.

Finally, a study published in 2017 in the renowned journal Nature (Molecular Psychiatry) demonstrates the interaction between **stress** and healthy nutrition: two groups of women thus followed either a pro- or anti-inflammatory diet, with measurement of their blood levels of markers of inflammation and their state of stress. And guess what? The results observed in relation to the diet were only those expected (i.e. pro- or anti-inflammatory) when the reported stress level was low. At high levels of stress, the type of diet had no influence, meaning that both groups had high levels of inflammation. In summary, nutrition is an important factor, but secondary to good stress management.

So, what you eat is important, but **how** you eat is just as important. Avoid overstimulation during meals (TV, smartphone, meetings, etc.) and use this time to (re)connect with your family, colleagues, or yourself. This will have far more beneficial effects on you than you might imagine, not least in silencing your internal saboteurs (see below).

Movement

Movement is another very important aspect as it is essential for good health and performance. With its 600 muscles, 200 bones and 360 different joints, your body is made to move, and the **modern sedentary lifestyle** is a real scourge.

What is less well known is that the most important thing is to **move often**, even a little. The difference in positive impact on health is much greater between someone who moves a little and someone who is sedentary, than between someone who moves a little and a great athlete. The effect inside the body can be likened to the difference between stagnant water and flowing water. The better the circulation, the better the oxygenation (and therefore energy production), and the better the elimination of waste products.

The ideal is to **walk** between 7,000 and 10,000 steps a day, spread out over the course of the day, to do at least one **muscle-strengthening** session a week (body-weight work, with elastic bands and/or additional loads) and to include **mobility** work on a regular basis. You can also add, for example, 30–90-minute cycling sessions for good cardio-respiratory capacity (preferably outdoors in a non-polluted environment). Moderate physical activity (e.g. 15-20 minutes' walking or 30-40 squats) has a particularly beneficial effect on glycemia (blood sugar levels) and fat storage, if done before or within an hour of meals.

A positive side-effect of movement is that it promotes better breathing, and hence better **oxygenation**, than when we are sedentary. When we are sitting, leaning forward, our diaphragm - the most important muscle in breathing - can't work with good amplitude, and we are less oxygenated. The diaphragm also becomes less supple and elastic under prolonged stress. This is not a threat to our survival, but to our energy and health, especially over the long term.

When it comes to energy, think of a wood fire. If you blow on the embers, the fire starts again. It's the effect of oxygen, and it has the same effect on you. If you start to feel drowsy, get up, go outside, take a few deep breaths of air and you'll immediately feel better.

On the health front, the 1931 Nobel Prize-winning scientist **Otto Warburg** demonstrated that cells deprived of oxygen clump together and form tumors. This work was confirmed by **Dr. Harry Goldblatt** in 1973. Could this be one of the causes of cancer in our society? Personally, I think it contributes to it.

Natural cycles

Nature operates to the rhythm of seasonal, lunar, and circadian cycles.

We saw the importance of the circadian rhythm in the "sleep and recovery" section.

Another important aspect for you ladies (and indirectly for your spouses) is the way you experience your **menstrual cycle**. In very simple terms, the aim of the cycle is to perpetuate the human species by mating at the right time, and then either to allow your offspring to develop, or to put everything back in order to give you another chance to do so. The cycle is divided into 4 phases with different durations and hormone production: the follicular phase (7-10 days), ovulation (3-4 days), the luteal phase (10-14 days) and menstruation (3-7 days). Depending on the phase, your nutritional needs will vary, as will, for example, your propensity to store fat. Your athletic abilities will also differ according to phase. I recommend the book "Woman Code" by **Alisa Vitti** for a more in-depth look at this subject and adapting your lifestyle to your menstrual cycle.

By the same token, being able to adapt your lifestyle to the rhythm of the seasons will be extremely beneficial to your health, your zest for life and your performance. For example, we have more energy in spring and summer, so use it wisely. Take better care of yourself and rest in autumn and winter. Eat local, seasonal fruit and vegetables, which are best suited to your current needs.

EMOTIONAL ENERGY

"Emotions can get in the way or get you on the way." Mavis Mazhura

If physical energy is responsible for your energy quantity (high or low), emotional energy is more likely to influence its **quality**, and hence the quality of your whole life. Emotions can be broadly classified as pleasant or unpleasant, with more or less intensity depending on your physical energy.

Emotions are often perceived as momentary reactions. In other words, an emotion is a piece of **information** that is felt at a given moment. For example, if someone cuts you off, you feel angry. If your child scores the winning goal, you feel proud. So, your body first creates an emotional vibration - for example, the vibration of happiness, sadness, anxiety or excitement. Then you start to feel the emotion, as well as the thoughts and physical sensations that accompany it. This process can last a second or much longer. Eventually, in a healthy emotional life cycle, you choose to let go of the emotion and move on.

The purpose of emotions is to inform us to move us into action, hence their name (e-motion, energy in motion). Unpleasant emotions are therefore very useful in the short term. The problem arises when they persist. Let's take an example: if you bring your hand too close to a hot stove, you're going to get burned and you will quickly withdraw your hand. If you didn't, you would burn it a lot more. Pain is a **signal** for quick action.

When you feel emotions that seem unpleasant, welcome them, identify them, and look for the message they are communicating. Use the table below to see whether it would be worth re-evaluating the meaning you give them (e.g. stress or excitement?).

Situation	Automatic thoughts	Emotions	Alternatives thoughts	Emotions
Describe a past situation	What were your thoughts?	What did you feel?	What more useful thoughts could you have had instead?	How do you feel about these new thoughts?
The last meeting with my boss	I'm going to be lectured again.	I feel stressed.	It is a good opportunity to get his opinion.	I am looking forward to the discussion.

If you are naturally anxious, you can set aside what is known as **worry time** (for example, 20 minutes) to worry on purpose. Divide the list of everything you are worried about into two columns: things you can do something about, and things you can't do anything about. For the first column, list the objectives to be achieved and the actions to be taken, being as specific as possible. If necessary, create a mind map (see chapter 4). Then put your stressful thoughts aside for the rest of the day. Just putting them down on paper will have a liberating effect.

What I can do something about	What I can't do anything about
I'm afraid of being cold in winter → buy wood for extra heating.	I am afraid of a new confinement.
I am worried about my finances → I can create a mind map with all my options.	I am worried about the death of a loved one.

Breathing techniques such as **cardiac coherence** (5 seconds of inhalation and 5 seconds of exhalation for 5 minutes 1 to 3 times a day) or **box breathing** (minimum 4 seconds of inhalation, full retention, exhalation, and empty retention) are sure to help you manage your emotions, especially if you practice them regularly.

Another effective technique for quick action is the **5-4-3-2-1 technique** where you scan your environment and list 5 things you can see, 4 things you can smell or touch, 3 things you can hear, 2 things you can smell and 1 thing you can taste.

I will talk more about emotions in chapter 5 (letting go).

MENTAL ENERGY

"Where focus goes, energy flows." Tony Robbins

Mental energy reflects your ability to **focus** on what you really want, to put your energy in the right place so to speak. This notion of focus is intimately linked to your **commitment, desire,** and **motivation** to change, evolve and progress.

Your focus - what you put your attention on - is therefore crucial. We have a natural tendency to focus on what is going wrong, simply for historical reasons of survival. You then have three options:

- do nothing and brood more and more, becoming a negative person who isolates himself more and more from others,
- understand the message your unconscious is giving you and take action to change what is bothering you,
- change your focus to something more useful and enjoyable,

provided you have something to do. There are many people today, including the very young, who lack a flame and a sense of purpose in their lives, and this is directly linked to the fourth form of energy.

Depending on the circumstances, you can focus your attention either

- **inwards** through practices such as breathing, yoga or mindfulness, or
- **outwards**, through activities such as cooking, gardening, or a walk in the forest (like Shinrin-Yoku, the forest baths we know from Japan), where you connect with external sensations such as the warmth of the sun or wind on your skin, contact with trees, the different textures of bark, etc.

On a very practical note, what can you do when you are plagued by negative thoughts, for example when you find yourself in a professional environment that doesn't suit you?

You won't be able to stop thinking about it as long as you are stimulated. Your objective will be either to act as quickly as possible to change the situation if you can, or to create a **diversion** in your mind to stop the negative spiral inside your body (stress hormones, muscular tension, etc.). You have about ten seconds before other negative thoughts add up. To distract yourself, you can take a few deep breaths, focus on your senses, hum a song, or think of a funny situation. Distracting thoughts is what smokers do when they take a cigarette break (in the very short term, smoking improves breathing). So, use the same strategy, but in a healthier way!

In keeping with the principle of Yin and Yang, to focus, which can be likened to zooming in on our objectives, it is also useful to combine **dezooming**. Take a few minutes to identify brown objects around you. Name them out loud. Now think back to what you saw that was blue. Look around again. You will see that there is a lot more blue than you picked up by focusing only on brown.

Bear in mind that one strategy (in this case, focus, zoom) is unlikely to work in all cases, and that activating your complementary strategy (in this case, wide vision, zoom out) will help you to unblock certain situations by opening up the field of possibilities and increasing the number of options at your disposal.

Similarly, activating your **peripheral vision** will help you relax and rebalance your nervous system (by acting on the parasympathetic branch).

SPIRITUAL ENERGY

"The meaning of life is to find your gift. The purpose of life is to give it away." Pablo Picasso

Our spiritual energy is our most powerful source of **motivation, perseverance**, and **direction**. It is directly linked to our passion and what we want to achieve, both for ourselves (our **ego**) and beyond ourselves (our **soul**). I am adopting here the definitions of ego and soul used by **Robert Dilts** in his series of books "Success Factor Modeling" because I find it very powerful to really work on these two axes (again the Yin and the Yang).

For example, people who are depressed tend to withdraw into themselves and neglect the altruistic aspect of the soul, which will further sink them. If this is your case, pay more attention to others (your family, your friends, your colleagues, people in need…) and you will quickly feel much better (also read the section on needs).

It is **passion** that gives extraordinary people the courage to start an ambitious project, whether it is personal, sports-related, scientific, or entrepreneurial, and the strength to persevere in difficult times. It is passion that drives you to wake up early and stay up late to achieve your dreams. It is passion that you desire in your relationships. There is no grand aspiration without passion!

We also find at the spiritual level the notions of

- **vision**: what we want to see differently in the world (for example, more people in better health),
- **mission**: how we can contribute to it (for example, by becoming a healthcare professional or an organic farmer), and
- **role**: who does what, a very important aspect when working in a team.

The more **clarity** you have on these different aspects, the more centered and **confident** you will feel in yourself and your abilities.

Viktor Frankl's texts on the power of spiritual capacity to transform even the most horrible circumstances into something positive are very moving. Frankl is a psychologist who survived the Nazi concentration camps and later wrote the classic "Man's Search for Meaning" where he quotes **Nietzsche**'s famous words: "He who has a 'why' to live can bear almost any 'how'."

According to him, mental health rests on a certain degree of tension, between what one has already accomplished and what one still should accomplish, or in other words, the gap between what one is and what one should become. What Man really needs is not a state without tension, but rather effort and struggle towards a **worthwhile goal**, through a **freely chosen task**.

SEXUAL ENERGY

Our sexual energy greatly influences our behavior towards others, especially in our romantic relationships.

Indeed, the interplay of **masculine** and **feminine polarities**, when truly present in a relationship, is what creates that "spark" of sexual energy. The more the sexual energies between two people are opposed, the stronger the attraction will be in the relationship. Physical attraction, spiritual ecstasy, and intimate connection flourish better in a relationship when there is a distinct sexual polarity between the energies of the two partners.

If two people have a similar sexual polarity, meaning they are both more "masculine" or more "feminine", the attraction between them will be less. On the other hand, if there is a strong difference, if one is extremely "feminine" and the other "masculine", the physical attraction will be maximal. This is the attraction of opposites in action.

Like Yin and Yang, they complement each other wonderfully if one is aware of them and activates them judiciously (since, I repeat, we all have these two types of energy, regardless of our gender and sexual orientation).

Any person, whether male or female, can embody either energy. People with **masculine energy** tend to be strong, problem-solvers within a mission framework (sense of purpose), and seek to break free from the constraints of life. They are competitive and may have difficulty expressing their emotions while wanting to feel appreciated in their relationships.

People with **feminine energy** are more open and free, ready to give and receive love. Feminine energies want to be noticed and understood, and their loving nature can lead them to stay in a relationship for too long.

The most important thing regarding sexual polarity is to know one's true nature and how it manifests. Some people may activate one much more than the other, sometimes at the expense of the other. The cause often comes from early childhood and the relationship with one or the other parent, resulting in relational dysfunctions that can be passed down from generation to generation. Fortunately, this can all be rebalanced through coaching or therapy.

If you are in a relationship, you can use this concept to strengthen it. Are you looking for love? When you accept and cultivate your innate energy, you naturally attract partners who complement you. Once you understand and accept the energy you emit, you will attract more of the opposite energy in return.

QUANTUM ENERGY

"Nothing is lost, nothing is created, everything is transformed." Antoine Lavoisier

While this book was being written, I came across "The Seeker's Code" by **Donny Epstein**, which had just been released.

In it, the author presents us with a version of energy that is more subtle, less consciously palpable, but nevertheless present. He introduces the **codes of creation** that organize our existence and what we manifest around us.

The codes of creation are the principles of **self-organization** that allow the manifestation of everything in the Universe. An example of this is the way a spider weaves its web; it needs neither an architect's plans nor a manual. These codes shape our bodies, our emotions, our ability to think, and our connection to the immaterial nature of life.

According to the author, all the data around us is energy, and what we manifest depends on the amount of energy we can express at any given moment. Energy is thus a **currency** (nothing is lost, nothing is created, everything is transformed) between all things, including ourselves and our environment. Our thoughts and emotions are energy.

Indeed, there is an **electromagnetic field** around us that is a force of **attraction** and **repulsion** for everything and everyone. It is this field that connects us all, somewhat like the internet. The way we interact optimally with it can be done in two different ways: either from the past to the future or from the future to the past. It is up to us to experiment to find the one that best suits us.

This work on energy is found in yoga and martial arts and is consistent with what has been presented about emotions. When certain emotions are trapped, they can indeed block certain chakras, energy centers found throughout the body, which according to ancient texts number 88,000. The 7 main ones (located along the spine) are connected to the major endocrine glands (the glands that produce stress, sexual, thyroid hormones, etc.). These glands could also be the source of our emotions, which also explains the link that Chinese medicine, for example, makes between emotions and organs.

Note that each main chakra is associated with a color, which is also a vibration. Choose carefully the colors you wear and those that decorate your home and/or office.

I will spare you the theoretical aspects of quantum physics that go beyond the scope of this book. Just keep in mind that if you realize that in certain circumstances, everything presented in this book does not work for you, it is this section that I would advise you to delve into, as I am currently doing personally.

Exercise: Evaluate your overall energy level. On a scale of 1 to 10 (1 representing the lowest value and 10 the highest), how would you rate your mastery of your 6 energies, and your ability to regenerate them? If you are above 8, that is great; refine your habits to move to the next level. If you are below 8, an action plan is necessary. Below 5, it is urgent!

To conclude this chapter, and still in connection with Yin and Yang, your success will depend both on your ability to **engage fully** and completely, and on your ability to **disengage strategically** when necessary (either when you need to recharge your batteries or when the game is not worth the candle).

FOR MORE INFORMATION

Awaken the Giant Within: How to Take Immediate Control of Your Mental, Emotional, Physical & Financial Destiny, Anthony Robbins, 1991

Boundless: Upgrade Your Brain, Optimize Your Body & Defy Aging, Ben Greenfield, 2020

Depression, Daily Stressors And Inflammatory Responses To High-Fat Meals : When Stress Overrides Healthier Food Choices. Kiecolt-Glaser et al, Molecular Psychiatry (2017) 22, 476-482 (https://nature.com/articles/mp2016149.epdf)

Earthing - Connexion à la Terre - Live avec Hugues Ostoja-Kuczynski, https://youtube.com/live/8k7ZSoVnyBM?feature=share

Et Si Votre Maison Troublait Votre Sommeil ? Hugues Ostoja-Kuczynski, 2020

Experiencing Physical Warmth Promotes Interpersonal Warmth, Lawrence E. Williams And John A. Bargh, Science, Vol 322 (24 Oct 2008), Issue 5901: 606-607

Life Force: How New Breakthroughs In Precision Medicine Can Transform The Quality Of Your Life & Those You Love, Tony Robbins, 2022

Man's Search for Meaning: The Classic Tribute to Hope from The Holocaust, Viktor Frankl, 2004

Mind Map Mastery: The Complete Guide to Learning and Using the Most Powerful Thinking Tool in The Universe, Tony Buzan, 2018

Neurotransmetteurs et Nutrition du Stress, https://www.pensersante.fr/neurotransmetteurs-nutrition-du-stress

On The Malignant Transformation Of Cells During Prolonged Culture Under Hypoxic Conditions *in vitro,* Harry Goldblatt, Libby Friedman, Ronald L. Cechner, Biochemical Medicine, Volume 7, Issue 2, April 1973, Pages 241-252, https://www.sciencedirect.com/science/article/abs/pii/0006294473900793

Positive Intelligence: Why Only 20% Of Teams And Individuals Achieve Their True Potential And How You Can Achieve Yours, Shirzad Chamine, 2012

Relations Amoureuses, Familiales ... Se Libérer Des Schémas De Souffrance, avec Franck Lopvet, https://youtu.be/GuoHRy8FBNU?si=MBk9nPeDK38K7nsX

The Body Code: Unlocking Your Body's Ability to Heal Itself, Bradley Nelson, 2023

The Emotion Code: How to Release Your Trapped Emotions for Abundant Health, Love, and Happiness (Updated and Expanded Edition), Bradley Nelson, 2019

The Functional Medicine Tree, Frank Lipman, https://youtu.be/DBdFq9O3W-8?si=_YrlMJgcwZlSmHuf

The Law of Polarity, Tony Robbins, https://www.tonyrobbins.com/ask-tony/polarity/

The Power of Full Engagement, Jim Loehr & Tony Schwartz, 2003

The Power of When: Discover Your Chronotype--and the Best Time to Eat Lunch, Ask for a Raise, Have Sex, Write a Novel, Take Your Meds, and More, Michael Breus, 2016

The Seeker's Code: Your Access to The Unreasonable and Extraordinary, Donny Epstein, 2023

Tout sur les Chakras ou Presque, Céline Miconnet, 2019, https://blog.green-yoga.fr/tout-sur-chakras-ou-presque/

Unlimited Power, Anthony Robbins, 1986

Voluntary Activation of The Sympathetic Nervous System and Attenuation of The Innate Immune Response in Humans. Kox et al, Proceedings of the National Academy of Sciences USA (2014) 111 (20) 7379-84 (https://ncbi.nlm.nih.gov/pubmed/24799686)

Wim Hof Method, https://www.wimhofmethod.com

Woman Code: Perfect Your Cycle, Amplify Your Fertility, Supercharge Your Sex Drive and Become a Power Source, Alisa Vitti, 2013

3 - MASTER YOUR MINDSET

"Your attitude, not your aptitude, will determine your altitude." Zig Ziglar

"Talent is not passed down in the genes. It is passed down in the mindset." Carol Dweck

"The empires of the future are empires of the mind." Winston Churchill

"Make an empire of your thoughts." Richard Francis Burton

If the previous chapter was more related to what is happening in your body, this one will focus more on what is happening inside your **head**.

American psychologist **Carol S. Dweck** has devoted her career to studying mindset, which she differentiates between a **fixed mindset** and a **growth mindset**. In her book "Mindset: The New Psychology of Success", she explains, with numerous examples from her research findings, anecdotes from everyday life, and biographical elements of famous personalities, how having a mindset oriented towards learning and continuous improvement (the growth mindset) leads to a much richer life in terms of success and fulfillment in all areas (education, social and romantic relationships, sports, business).

Do you think your intelligence is an innate trait that you can't really change? Do you believe you cannot change essential components of your personality? If you answered "yes", you most likely have a fixed mindset. If, on the contrary, you believe that, regardless of your level of intelligence, you can improve it, and change certain aspects of your personality, then you definitely have a growth mindset.

Skills and talent alone are not enough. The most important thing to face and overcome challenges is to approach them with a growth mindset. As you may have guessed, to make the impossible possible, this is the mindset you will need.

Michael Jordan wasn't a natural born athlete, but he was one of the hardest workers in the history of sports. He was cut from his high school varsity basketball team, not recruited by the University of North Carolina, his dream school, and not drafted by the first two NBA teams that could have picked him. When he was cut from the varsity team, he was devastated. But he got in the habit of leaving home at 6am to practice before school. At the University of North Carolina, he constantly worked on his weaknesses. Even at the height of his glory, his relentless training was legendary. For him, success comes from the mindset. Champions are not born, they are made.

Of course, we all have both mindsets, perhaps one more than the other, and perhaps differently depending on the areas of our lives (health, finances, love, work...).

Mindset can be defined as everything that influences your way of thinking, especially:

- your needs,
- your representation of the world,
- your past experiences,
- your beliefs,
- your confidence in yourself,
- your language,
- your self-discipline and
- your decisions.

YOUR NEEDS

There are many theories aimed at explaining why we do what we do. The simplest and most powerful one I know, and personally use in my coaching, is **Tony Robbins'** six human needs approach. It also helps to better understand our **emotions** for better relationships and thus a better quality of life.

Indeed, it is emotions that drive you to action, hence their name (energy in motion, E-motion). Overall, we all seek to move towards **pleasure** and away from **pain**.

According to **Tony Robbins**, there are 6 universal human needs that you absolutely must satisfy to achieve this goal:

- **certainty**: the assurance of avoiding pain and gaining pleasure (other names can be used such as routine, security, control),
- **uncertainty**: the need for the unknown, change, variety, new stimuli,
- **significance**: the need to feel unique, important, special, or necessary,
- **love and connection**: the need for a strong sense of closeness or bond with someone or something,
- **growth**: the need for the expansion of capabilities, skills, or understanding, and
- **contribution**: the need to have a sense of service and to focus on helping, giving, and supporting others.

When your needs are not met, you experience unpleasant emotions:

- **anxiety** when you lack certainty,
- **boredom** when you lack variety,
- **low self-esteem** or **contempt from others** when you lack significance,
- **loneliness** when you lack love and connection,
- **frustration** when you lack growth,
- **emptiness** or lack of meaning when you lack contribution.

Humans are resourceful and can find many means (**vehicles**) to satisfy their needs; some are healthy, and some are not, as we often seek immediate gratification instead of thinking long-term.

Take the importance, for example: you can feel important by constantly talking about yourself or belittling others, or you can satisfy this need by developing yourself and bringing value to others.

The need for connection can be satisfied by creating meaningful relationships and helping others, or by smoking, drinking, or overeating (connecting with oneself).

In reality, things are often much more nuanced, but you get what I mean.

These vehicles should ideally be linked to your **values**. These are fundamental judgments of an ethical, moral, or practical nature that you hold about what really matters to you, what is valuable to you in essence. They constitute a set of beliefs about what you consider right or wrong in your life, and reasons you give yourself to believe that life is worth living. Many people do not have a clear idea of what they consider important. On the other hand, successful people always have a very clear vision of what they consider important. You will find an exercise in the "Tools" section of Chapter 4 to determine your values and identify those to add or reprioritize.

Once the vehicles are identified, it is interesting to think about the **rules** to follow. Suppose you want to nourish your need for growth by growing your business (your vehicle). What do you need to be satisfied: 10% more customers? 1000% more? If you want to reduce your body fat to feel more important, at what percentage will you be satisfied? 25? 10?

The stricter your rules are, the harder it will be for you to be happy. A healthy way to proceed is to **gradually raise the bar** higher and higher instead of focusing solely on unattainable goals.

When something or someone simultaneously meets at least three of our needs, we can consider it an **addiction**. Think, for example, of overeating. It gives you (i) the certainty of feeling good in the short term (relaxing effect of digestion that activates the parasympathetic branch), (ii) the variety of the state you want to change, and (iii) the connection with yourself. The same goes for smokers, with the additional connection with others when they gather at the "smokers" corner.

As I mentioned earlier, we will do whatever it takes to meet our needs (especially the first four). This can even go as far as violating our own values. For example, a woman who had been married for a long time had a lover and felt guilty because her behavior went against her values. Yet she could not choose between the two men because her husband met her needs for certainty and love, while her lover fulfilled her needs for variety and significance.

Now that you know the 6 human needs and the emotions you feel when they are not met, you have probably identified the 2 needs that are most important to you. These 2 **primary needs** determine your life. If you give more importance to certainty than anything else, your life will be completely different than if you prioritize love first.

We all have the six needs, and all are important, but the ranking matters more in terms of joy and fulfillment. So, if you want to change your life, focus more on love, growth, and contribution.

If you are in a **relationship**, try to meet your needs and those of your partner based on each other's respective vehicles and rules. Also, keep in mind that you are responsible for meeting your own needs and not just wait for the other person to do it for you.

YOUR REPRESENTATION OF THE WORLD

Our world is a kaleidoscope of **sensory experiences**. Every day, we are inundated with a multitude of visual, auditory, tactile, olfactory, and gustatory information, even more so today than yesterday.

But how does our mind process all this data to create a coherent **perception** of the external world that we know? In fact, we do not all perceive the same situation in the same way, which can generate misunderstandings and even conflicts.

Your **senses** are your gateways to the external world. They allow you to capture crucial information about your environment. Vision provides you with an overview of the world, hearing enables you to hear sounds and music, touch connects you to the texture and temperature of objects, smell informs you about scents, and taste allows you to savor the diversity of flavors. Each of these senses plays an essential role in how you perceive the external world.

As your brain cannot process everything at once, it consciously and unconsciously selects sensory information. There are thus **information losses** that will be different from one person to another (which can cause misunderstanding and conflicts). This selection often depends on your attention (recall the exercise of the brown and blue colors), your past experiences, and your motivations.

You can use this specificity to your advantage by **visualizing** as clearly as possible what you want to achieve and/or obtain (and by visualizing it in the most sensory way possible, as if it had already happened).

Indeed, you activate your **reticular activating system** (RAS), an anatomical structure in the brain that plays a crucial role in regulating the state of wakefulness and vigilance. It is located in the brainstem, a region of the brain at the base of your skull and extends into the posterior brain. The RAS is responsible for maintaining alertness, attention, and overall vigilance, and plays a key role in filtering sensory stimuli and modulating brain activity based on the perceived importance of incoming information. Think of a small white car and you will notice more on the road. It is not because there are suddenly a lot more, it is just that your RAS will filter the numerous sensory information you receive constantly, prioritizing certain information for cognitive processing while ignoring others. This helps to avoid information overload. The RAS also regulates the activity of different brain regions according to needs. For example, it can increase the activity of regions involved in problem-solving when a cognitive task requires deep thinking.

Your brain does not passively process sensory information; it also organizes it to create a **coherent perception** of the world. This means that what you perceive is not a mere copy of reality, but rather a mental construct based on your senses, beliefs, and expectations.

Optical illusions are a fascinating example of this. They show how our brain can be deceived by visual configurations that contradict reality. This reminds us that perception is often a subjective interpretation of the external world.

Our perceptions are influenced by a series of **cognitive biases**. Among the most common are:

- **confirmation bias**, where we tend to notice and remember information that confirms our preexisting beliefs.
- **availability bias**, where we give more importance to information that is easily accessible in our memory.
- **selection bias**, where we filter information to favor those that match our interests or point of view.

Awareness of these biases is essential for a more objective perception of the external world. By recognizing that your perception is often subjective and influenced by multiple factors, you can become more open to **new perspectives** and more tolerant of viewpoints different from your own.

Thus, it is not so much what happens to you that matters, but the representation you make of it. Two children walking on the beach and getting splashed by a wave can react very differently; one may start crying and run to their mother, and the other may have fun and shout "Again!". The most effective business leaders, athletes, and parents are those who succeed in representing events in a positive way despite discouraging signs, both to themselves and to others, and thus continue to act until they succeed.

Obviously, this ability to stay positive depends on your ability to put yourself in a **favorable state**, hence the importance of energy management as seen in the previous chapter. Everything is interconnected.

Finally, as we do not all perceive things with the same sensory preferences (mainly visual, auditory, and kinesthetic), excellent **communication** will involve identifying the other person's preferential channels (which may be different from yours, which is most likely the case with people you get along less well with) and adapting your message accordingly. If your boss is primarily visual, you will not convince them through speech but rather through text or a diagram.

YOUR PAST EXPERIENCES

We all carry, often without realizing it, an **invisible baggage** filled with our past experiences. These experiences, whether joyful or painful, contribute to shaping your **identity**, your **choices**, and your **vision of the future**.

Your **memory** is the storage place for your past experiences. It records the events, emotions, and lessons you have drawn from your life. Your memories, whether conscious or buried in your subconscious, shape both your perception of the present and the future.

However, memory is not just a simple archive. It is **subject to biases, distortion**, and **selective forgetting**. We often remember selectively, favoring emotionally impactful experiences or information that confirms our existing beliefs. For example, if you have experienced repeated failures in a particular area, you may develop negative beliefs about your skills in that area. Conversely, positive experiences can reinforce your self-confidence and positive beliefs.

Your past experiences also create patterns of **behavior** that can become **habits**. For example, if you learned to cope with stress by emotionally eating during childhood, this can become a behavioral pattern that you reproduce in adulthood during times of stress.

These patterns of behavior can be beneficial or harmful, and they are often **unconscious**. Becoming aware of them is the first step in bringing about positive changes in your life.

Indeed, although your past experiences may partly shape you, they do not condemn you to an immutable fate. Reflection and healing are powerful tools for understanding and transforming their impact. **Reflection** involves stepping back to examine your experiences, beliefs, and behavioral patterns. This can be done through meditation, therapy, writing, discussion with others, or coaching. **Healing** involves working on resolving your traumas, emotional wounds, and destructive behavior patterns. This may involve seeking help from a mental health professional.

Ultimately, your past experiences are a real source of **opportunities** for your personal growth. The challenges you have overcome, the lessons you have learned, and the moments of joy you have experienced all contribute to your development as human beings.

Understanding how your past experiences have shaped you will help you make more informed decisions, reduce self-destructive behaviors, and create a more fulfilling life. It is a deeply personal journey, but it can be one of the most rewarding you have ever undertaken.

In **mental training**, one of the strategies is to put yourself in a particular mental state to project yourself into the future to create the experience that you want to see happen in the future as if it were happening right now because our brain does not distinguish between reality and imagination. This is called the **anticipated experience of results** and is one of the many benefits of imagination.

YOUR BELIEFS

"Believe you can and you are halfway there." Theodore Roosevelt

Your beliefs are one of the invisible **foundations** upon which you build your reality. If they are solid and deeply rooted, your mental empire will withstand the storms of doubt and uncertainty. If they are fragile, even the slightest shake can bring down your inner world.

A belief is a **deep conviction**, a sense of **inner certainty** about something that often is not immediately perceptible by our senses. It is a conviction that something is true, even in the absence of tangible evidence.

Beliefs are pre-established **filters** through which we perceive the world. They encompass everything from our faith in a god, a scientific theory, a system of values, to our confidence in our own ability to succeed. They primarily come from our environment and our past experiences.

When you firmly believe that something is true, it is as if you are giving your brain an order on how to represent events to you. If you believe that the world is a dangerous place, your daily experience will be tinged with mistrust and fear. If you believe that life is beautiful and full of possibilities, you will be more open and inclined to see opportunities and live with optimism.

But beliefs are not just filters through which you perceive the outside world, they also influence your **inner world**. They dictate your thoughts, your emotions, your actions, and thus your results. If you believe you are destined to fail, your actions will reflect that belief, unconsciously sabotaging you at every turn. Conversely, if you believe in your unlimited potential, you will be more inclined to pursue your dreams with determination and perseverance.

Your beliefs are the force that determines:

-   what you try or do not try to accomplish in your life,
-   what is possible or impossible,
-   what you are capable of and
-   who you are.

Think of the **placebo effect**, where a medicine devoid of any healing properties acts on the patient who is convinced that they are being given an effective treatment. Did you know that it can be effective in 30 to 60% of people?

Beliefs are also contagious, influencing those around you. Your faith in something can inspire others to share that conviction. It can also lead to disagreements when your beliefs conflict with those of others. Nonetheless, understanding the importance of beliefs can help you build bridges rather than walls.

Your beliefs are not set in stone. They evolve over time as you acquire new knowledge and experiences and as you reassess your perspectives. However, it is essential to be aware of your beliefs, to examine them closely, and to consciously decide which ones you want to keep and develop and which ones you want to let go of.

<u>Exercise</u>: What are the major beliefs you have about yourself and what you can achieve? List 5 limiting beliefs from your past and 5 beliefs that can help you achieve your most ambitious dreams.

YOUR SELF-CONFIDENCE

"Believe in your dreams and they may come true. Believe in yourself and they will surely come true." Martin Luther King

Your self-confidence is one of the most precious jewels you can cultivate in your life. It is closely linked to your **self-esteem** (the value you place on yourself), your **skills**, and your **relationship with others**.

Imagine self-confidence as an imposing **wall**. Each brick that makes it up is a belief you hold about yourself. These beliefs are shaped by your history, experiences, interactions with others, and, of course, your inner thoughts.
If you believe in your intrinsic worth as a human being, if you believe in your ability to learn and grow, then your wall of self-confidence soars high into the sky. You feel capable of taking on any challenge, overcoming any difficulty. You have faith in yourself.

However, if your beliefs are filled with doubts and self-criticism, then your wall of self-confidence will be weakened. You will hesitate to take risks, pursue your dreams, or assert yourself in your relationships.

The connection between your **beliefs** and your self-confidence is deeply symbiotic. Your beliefs influence your level of confidence, and your confidence, in turn, reinforces or challenges your beliefs. It is a cycle that can be either virtuous or vicious.

When you recognize this link, you have the power to deliberately reshape it. You can examine your limiting beliefs and replace them with positive and constructive beliefs. This may require inner work, deep reflection, and sometimes even the help of a professional. But the result is worth it.

Self-confidence is not arrogance. It does not involve believing you are superior to others. On the contrary, it is a **profound humility** that stems from self-awareness. It allows you to recognize your strengths and weaknesses, to accept them, and to use them to the best of your abilities.

In short, your self-confidence and your beliefs are powerful allies in your quest to make the impossible possible, or simply to live a fulfilling life. By understanding the close link that unites them, you can build a solid wall of self-confidence capable of withstanding challenges and lifting you to new heights.

Self-confidence is not reserved for a select few. It is **accessible to all** and can be forged and strengthened through what is presented in this book.

YOUR LANGUAGE

"No matter what people tell you, words and ideas can change the world." Robin Williams

The words you use, whether aloud or in your inner monologue, are of **paramount importance**, both for yourself and for those who hear you.

An "excellent" meal doesn't have the same flavor as a dish that is "not too bad". Firstly, because it is much more powerful to speak without negation (our subconscious doesn't perceive it, so it mainly receives "bad" in the example above) and secondly, because what we associate with "excellent" is much stronger than what we associate with "good". For several years now, I have made it a habit to replace "have a nice day" with "have a beautiful day" or "wonderful day to you". Give it a try and you will feel the difference.

You can easily (and for free) **amplify your positive sensations** just by changing the words you use.

This is also true when describing an unpleasant situation. "I am furious" does not resonate the same way as "I am upset".

Exercise: Take the time to write down the 5-10 positive words you use the most. Do the same with the negative ones. Then look for other words, either more positive or less negative, with which you can replace them. Keep the list in sight to remind yourself to use these new words regularly and see what changes it brings. You will be surprised!

I really want to emphasize the power we have over others, especially the young ones (including our children). The words we use are not only the ones they hear, but very likely the ones they will use themselves. So, let's be more than vigilant!

Beyond simple words, **metaphors** have even more power. A metaphor consists of a modification of meaning (concrete term in an abstract context) by analogical substitution. We use it to describe something in an imaginative way with a different meaning. For example, "I feel like I am carrying the weight of the world on my shoulders" or "I feel as light as a feather". Repeat each of these phrases out loud. What do you feel? It is different, isn't it?

How would you describe your life? A game? An exciting adventure? A journey through the desert? A torment? And what would your ideal life be like? And what if that became your new metaphor from today?

The **questions** you ask yourself are also very important. Asking yourself better questions will lead to better answers. "Why does this only happen to me?" will not generate the same feelings, ideas, and responses as "What can I do to improve the situation?" and "Who can help me achieve this more quickly and easily?".

Asking yourself better questions will also help you develop your **critical thinking** and thus better differentiate what and who you can trust. In a world where information is omnipresent (we now even talk about information overload), being able to distinguish the true from the false has become an essential quality.

Questions are also a wonderful means of **communication** (which is why they are a major tool in coaching, which I particularly appreciate). Instead of giving your opinion, even if it is with kindness, take an interest in the other person by asking them a question. And as with everything in this book, don't just take my word for it, try it out for yourself!

Then there is that famous little voice in your head, responsible for your **inner monologue**. What does it tell you? Does it urge you to persevere? To be creative? To be happy or sad? It is likely to be naturally more negative for survival's sake. But we all have the power to control it! It will certainly require some effort (just like maintaining good personal hygiene) but it is well worth the effort!

Take the time to be more attentive to it in various circumstances and see how you can improve it to your advantage. Here is a tip: talk to yourself in "you" as if you were hearing the voice of a coach: "You will make it", "Be patient", "Stand tall"... A study led by **James Hardy** and his collaborators in 2019 demonstrated that it was more effective in terms of performance than speaking in the first person or neutrally.

In some cases, the most useful thing will be to simply tell it to shut up and quickly act. **Tony Robbins** has made it a habit to plunge into an ice-cold bath every morning, not only for the benefits to the body but also to condition his nervous system to shut up and obey when necessary.

Finally, I will end this section by talking about the importance of mantras. A **mantra** is a sacred formula, a short prayer, an incantation, and by extension, a phrase or idea that is constantly repeated. The more you repeat it, the more it will be ingrained in you.

Exercise: Create your own mantra, for example, "I am getting better and better every day" and display it in sight. Repeat it regularly, especially when you wake up and before going to bed, or when you doubt or go through a difficult period. You can even include it in your meditation practices, emphasizing each word for a longer time and feeling/seeing/hearing what it generates in you. Also, let it evolve over time if necessary.

YOUR SELF- DISCIPLINE

"Through discipline comes freedom." Aristotle

Self-discipline, also known as **willpower** or **determination**, is one of the things that sets us apart from animals, as the entire process of self-discipline takes place in the prefrontal cortex of the brain, which is much larger in humans compared to other mammals with the same brain structure. It allows humans to plan and analyze other possible actions instead of just doing what they want.

It is the ability to resist immediate temptations to achieve a greater reward in the long term. It is the **inner strength** that drives you to persevere when obstacles arise in your path.

It is also the ability to eliminate any unwanted feeling, thought, or impulse, especially when going through a difficult period.

Willpower, or self-discipline, thus has three different aspects:

- the ability to do what needs to be done (**"I must"**),
- the awareness of your desires and personal goals (**"I want to"**), and
- the ability to resist impulses and temptations (**"I do not want to"**).

You must use these three elements not only to **achieve your goals** but also to **avoid problems**.

Self-discipline is a form of conscious effort and self-regulation to resist temptations, control impulses, and maintain control.

Your self-discipline largely depends on your **habits**. Indeed, it is the choices you make at every moment, the small actions you take day after day, that shape your character and determine your results and ultimately your destiny.

If you cultivate self-discipline, you can turn the impossible into the possible, as there is an undeniable link between self-discipline and success. The most accomplished individuals in all areas of life are often those who have mastered the art of self-discipline by being able to set clear goals, follow an action plan, and persevere in the face of setbacks.

Your self-discipline is also directly connected to your **personal standards**, rules, and personal guidelines that help you in your actions and in making daily decisions. The higher your standards, the more discipline they demand. If you want to improve your self-discipline and the overall quality of your life, you must **raise the bar** and set higher personal standards. It is like making a deal with yourself. You have a list of things you allow yourself to do and others that you forbid yourself from doing. Consider gradually and continuously raising your standards for better long-term results.

You can also use **rewards** and **punishments** to encourage good behavior. Your levels of motivation can sometimes increase or decrease depending on various factors.

There will be times when you are on a roll and accomplish much more than you are supposed to. If you are in such a dynamic, you can reward yourself, for example, by indulging yourself for the rest of the day once your important tasks are completed.

On the other hand, if you have wasted your time on unnecessary things, you can penalize yourself by working longer the next day or depriving yourself of a pleasant moment that you had planned.

Finally, practice **self-compassion** in addition to self-discipline (the Yin and the Yang, remember?). Learn to forgive yourself for your failures to continue moving forward and improving.

YOUR DECISIONS

"Stay committed to your decisions, but stay flexible in your approach." Tony Robbins

Sometimes making the impossible possible comes down to a single decision. When in 1955 **Rosa Parks** boarded a bus in Montgomery, Alabama, and refused to give up her seat to a white man as the law required, she had no idea of the consequences. This single act of civil disobedience sparked a violent controversy. It was the beginning of the civil rights movement and became **a symbol for future generations.**

Every day of our lives is punctuated with decisions. Some will be more trivial (or not), such as choosing what clothes to wear, while others will have much more impact, such as deciding to change jobs or move to another country.

I recently discussed this with a retired business owner for whom the impact of past decisions was still very much present. Indeed, every choice we make can leave an indelible mark on ourselves or others, whether it is emotional, financial, legal, or otherwise.

Your decisions are also **interconnected**. Indeed, every choice you make can influence others. For example, the decision to pursue additional training can influence the career you choose, your income, your place of residence, and even your personal relationships. It is surprising to see that a seemingly insignificant decision can, through a domino effect, lead to an extraordinary result. I increasingly enjoy looking back and "**connecting the dots**", as **Steve Jobs** used to say. You would be surprised to know what simple decision to send an email triggered a cascade of positive events in my personal life.

The quality of your decisions largely depends on your ability to be **honest** and **congruent** with yourself, to step back, evaluate your options, draw from your past experiences, and anticipate future consequences. Knowing how to make better decisions is therefore an important skill to develop.

The first step is to **clarify** your goals, values, and priorities. Understanding what is truly important to you will help filter what is most in harmony with your true essence. For example, if family is one of your core values, a professional decision that would require a move away from loved ones deserves deeper thought and discussion with those involved.

Next, it is essential to **gather relevant information**. The more you know about your options, the better your decisions will be. This may involve research, consulting experts, or seeking advice from trusted individuals.

Decision-making also requires a dose of **courage**. Sometimes you have to make difficult decisions that involve sacrifices or risks. However, it is often in these moments of courage that the most rewarding **opportunities** are found.

The decision-making process is also **dynamic**. You must be prepared to reassess your choices and adjust when necessary. Your needs and constraints change over time, and your decisions must reflect these changes.

Continuous learning is one of the keys to making better decisions. Be open to feedback, whether positive or negative. If a decision does not yield the expected results, it does not necessarily mean failure, but rather an opportunity to learn and do better next time... or simply to have taken another step in the desired direction.

In summary, your decisions are somewhat your **superpowers**. Use them wisely.

FOUR POWERFUL MINDSETS OF KARATE

"Karate aims to develop the character, sincerity, and commitment of its practitioners." Kenji Tomiki

The mindset is particularly important in karate and martial arts in general, where the practice of the **path** demands special moral and personal qualities. Here are 4 mindsets of karate that can inspire you.

- **Shoshin**: the beginner's mind

When practicing martial arts and visiting another school, it is customary to wear a white belt, even if you are more advanced, in order to adopt this beginner's mindset. Indeed, a beginner will have a greater **open-mindedness** and be more receptive to learning than an expert who may be more set in their ways.

In the context of martial arts and in a personal defense situation, it will be useful to have automatism for greater effectiveness. However, in terms of learning, it will be more beneficial to have the broadest possible vision and not to limit yourself by your biases or personal filters. Each person sees the world with different lenses, based on the events they have experienced, the beliefs they have established, etc.

Putting yourself in this beginner's mindset is, in a way, wanting to eliminate all these lenses and look at the world around you with **pure eyes**.

- **Mushin**: the mind of no mind

This mindset may seem a bit strange at first. Let's say it corresponds to the state of **flow**, when you are so absorbed in what you are doing that you don't realize how time passes.

To be in this zone, you need to be able to do an activity that requires an appropriate level of effort based on your current abilities because if it is too easy, you get bored, and if it is too difficult, you can't do it, you get frustrated, etc.

To make it a little challenging and fun, the challenge should be slightly above your abilities. If it is also something you love to do, you will have an added sense of enjoyment.

However, you can get into this flow state even for a task you don't like, which will also be a question of **self-discipline**.

- **Fudoshin**: the immovable mind

This mindset corresponds to the notion of (total) **commitment**. When you have a goal with significant stakes, how much can you stay focused and committed to what you are doing?

It is somewhat related to Mushin since you will be more engaged when you are in a state of flow.

There will be moments when persisting, not giving up, will help you achieve your goal. And then at other times, if you find yourself facing a wall, it will be useless to keep hitting it. It will be more useful to step back and strategically disengage.

- **Zanshin**: the mind of consciousness

In a self-defense context, the idea is to know how to stay on your guard to anticipate aggression. In everyday life, it is also about being attentive to the **risks** and **dangers** that may arise around you in all areas, especially professionally.

It is also the ability to identify and seize opportunities when they arise. We live in an increasingly VUCA (Volatile, Uncertain, Complex, Ambiguous) world where risks, dangers, and **opportunities** are increasingly intertwined.

FOR MORE INFORMATION

Atomic Habits: An Easy & Proven Way to Build Good Habits & Break Bad Ones, James Clear, 2018

Awaken the Giant Within: How to Take Immediate Control of Your Mental, Emotional, Physical & Financial Destiny, Anthony Robbins, 1991

Four Powerful Mindsets of Karate, Jesse Enkamp, https://youtu.be/QjZ3IhHqBY8?si=1D_f3eS4d6qXs_bM

Giant Steps: Small Changes to Make a Big Difference, Tony Robbins, 1994

L'effet Placebo En Toute Transparence, Kheira Bettayeb, 2023, https://lejournal.cnrs.fr/articles/leffet-placebo-en-toute-transparence

Mindset: The New Psychology of Success, Carol S. Dweck, 2007

Peak: How all of us can achieve extraordinary things, Anders Ericsson & Robert Pool, 2017

Self-Discipline: The Spartan and Special Operations Way to Mastering Yourself, Ryan Hunt, 2019

The Big Leap: Conquer Your Hidden Fear and Take Life to The Next Level, Gay Hendricks, 2010

The Genius of Athletes: What World-Class Competitors Know That Can Change Your Life, Noel Brick & Scott Douglas, 2021

The Power of Mindset Change: Why Mindset Matters Most, Robert B Dilts & Mickey Feher, 2023

To Me, To You: How You Say Things Matters for Endurance Performance, James Hardy, Aled V. Thomas, and Anthony W. Blanchfield, Journal of Sports Sciences 37, no 18 (September 2019): 2122-30.

Unlimited Power, Anthony Robbins, 1986

Why We Do What We Do, Tony Robbins, 2006, TED talk, https://www.ted.com/talks/tony_robbins_why_we_do_what_we_do

4 - MASTER YOUR PERFORMANCE

"We gain strength, courage and confidence in the doing."
Theodore Roosevelt

"To become successful, you must be a person of action. Merely to 'know' is not sufficient. It is necessary both to know and do." Napoleon Hill

"The path to success is to take massive determined action." Tony Robbins

"I will prepare and some day my chance will come." Abraham Lincoln

OBJECTIVES

"Those who have no goals are unlikely to achieve them." Sun Tzu

Richie McCaw dreamed of being part of the All Blacks, the legendary New Zealand international rugby team.

Knowing that in New Zealand there are over 150,000 registered rugby players, about 3% of the population (compared to 1% in other countries), the goal was far from a sure thing.

When Richie shared his dreams with his uncle **John McLay**, he made him think about the steps to take to achieve his long-term ambition. Sitting in a restaurant one afternoon in 1998 (McCaw was 18 at the time), they both put on paper (a napkin to be precise) a series of career steps, with the goal of becoming an All Black by 2004.

But why stop there? McLay challenged the teenager to **aim even higher**, to become not just a "mere" All Black, but one of the greatest players to ever represent his country.

Richie made his debut with the All Blacks in 2001, against Ireland, 3 years before the planned date. Before retiring in 2015, after an international career of 148 matches, he was voted the best rugby player of the year three times. He also recorded the most victories and the most matches as captain. He is widely considered the greatest All Black of all time.

His progress highlights the principle of setting goals that most of us overlook, but to which many high-performing athletes adhere: **writing them down**. Recording your short and long-term goals will help you **focus** and **navigate**, especially when things don't go as hoped. McCaw's progress was not as smooth and linear as this condensed version of his story might suggest, but he stayed the course during the storms.

There are **different types of goals** that it is interesting to be able to distinguish:

- **outcome** goals (e.g. losing weight),
- **performance** goals (e.g. losing 10 kg),
- **process** goals (e.g. eating vegetables twice a day),
- **learning** goals (knowing the glycemic index of fruits), and
- **mastery** goals (improving from your personal standards - mastering the task at hand and developing your own skills and abilities to the highest possible level).

Most people have goals such as paying their bills, getting through their day, and surviving day after day, trapped in having to make a living rather than carving out a custom one. This kind of goal will not allow you to tap into the full potential that lies within you.

Instead, set goals that are big enough to go **beyond your limits**. Remember that while having a smartphone seems natural today, it did not exist thirty years ago. It even seemed impossible at the time to imagine talking to someone on the other side of the world via video conference. Someone had to invent it, and before inventing it, it had to be imagined with precision.

Take the time to reflect on your current situation in key areas of your life (e.g. health and physical appearance, romantic relationships, friendships, finances, career, etc.), that of 5 years ago (and celebrate your evolution), and then project yourself into 10 years. If at some point you feel discouraged, stopping and taking the time to savor the journey traveled will soothe your heart and allow you to make the necessary adjustments to continue moving forward.

In summary, have a mix of **SMART** (Specific, Measurable, Achievable, Realistic, and Time-bound) goals and others, much more open and **ambitious**, where you aim high, like becoming the greatest All Black of all time.

Exercise: List the goals you want to achieve (be as specific as possible). Then, fill in the following table with the experiences you want to live, how you need to develop to get there, and how you want to contribute around you. The 3 can be directly related or not.

Experience	Growth	Contribution
Live in California for 6 months	Learn English	Teach French in the USA
Play soccer in Division 1	Read biographies of famous players	Become a member of a service club

PLANIFICATION

"He who fails to plan is planning to fail." Sir Winston Churchill

Another inspiring story is that of **Richard Williams**, the tireless father of two of the most extraordinarily gifted athletes of all time, who changed the world of tennis forever.

The movie "King Richard", released in 2021 starring **Will Smith,** deeply moving in the role of **Richard Williams**, shows us the power of family, perseverance, and unwavering faith to achieve the impossible and impact the world.

Driven by a **clear vision of their future** and using unconventional methods, Richard created a plan that took **Venus and Serena Williams** from the streets of Compton, California, to the global stage, becoming legendary icons.

As seen in the two examples above, **Richie McCaw** and the **Williams family**, it is more effective to **break down major goals into smaller objectives** that will serve as milestones to both guide you and strengthen your confidence and perseverance. When defining short or medium-term actions, be as specific as possible. This will subtly facilitate your action. For example, if you need to go to the garage for maintenance on your car, your first action will be to make a phone call to schedule an appointment. By defining it in such clear terms, you will reduce your mental load and be much more inclined to make the call when you have a few minutes free.

As we will see in the "success strategy" section, the "if…then" technique will also be useful for planning the unforeseen. Then, the habits you put in place, and with what skill, will do the rest.

PRINCIPLES

"Success is more permanent when you achieve it without destroying your principles." Walter Cronkite

Principles will be very useful to give you a **guideline** for your life and get you closer to your goals. I am sharing with you 3 that I use very regularly for their power. Feel free to create your own. However, keep in mind **Bruce Lee**'s quote: "Respect the principles without being bound by them."

1. Take the most globale approach possible

According to **Arthur Koestler**, we are a **holon**, something that is both a whole and a part of a whole. Therefore, we must consider the widest possible perspective, knowing that what we neglect today could be our hindrance or problem tomorrow, if not already the case today.

On an individual level, consider both your **body** and your **mind**. Take care of your nutrition, your recovery, how you hold yourself and move, your thoughts, your emotions, your relationships, etc.

Within your family, make sure to include everyone according to their specificities.

In your professional environment (especially if you are a leader), also make sure to include as many perspectives as possible and ensure that all the gears are working optimally.

2. Apply the strategy of + and -

Here is an extremely simple principle and yet so underutilized! When aiming for a goal, consider what can bring you closer to it (the +) and what can take you away from it (the -). Then make the necessary adjustments by doing more of + and less (or even none) of -. This principle is directly related to your **habits**, hence the importance of being able to establish new beneficial habits and reduce or get rid of those that do not serve you (anymore). I will share more details on this topic a little further down.

3. Test and customize

We are all different, especially in terms of goals, abilities, and constraints. What is excellent for me may be very harmful for you.

Keep in mind that only a real test can demonstrate the effectiveness of a new action for you. This is especially true at the nutritional level, where the ideal proportions of fats and carbohydrates will vary, for example, depending on your neurotype (your neurotransmitter profile).

Remember to take note of the tests you carry out and **measure** the effects produced. Over time, you will build the **ideal system** for yourself.

STRATEGIES OF SUCCESS

Some strategies, when applied, inevitably lead to success. I will share 6 of them below.

1. The HIME

You probably know **Pareto**'s law, which states that 20% of our actions produce 80% of our results.

HIME (High Impact Minimal Effort) is about identifying and implementing activities that will have the most positive impact with minimal effort. Think of it as Pareto's law taken to the extreme (the 20% of the 20% of the 20%...).

By accumulating high-value-added activities, the **impact** can quickly become considerable.

Of course, it is not always possible to achieve high impact quickly (especially if the HIMEs have already been put in place). The following strategy then becomes very important.

2. The strategy of marginal gains

When **Dave Brailsford** joined the British cycling federation in 2003, its record was rather meager, with only one Olympic medal since 1908 and no victories in the famous Tour de France, one of the most legendary cycling races.

The performance of the British cycling team was so disappointing that one of the best European bicycle manufacturers had refused to sell them their machines, fearing a negative impact on sales.

Brailsford's goal was clear: to reverse the trend. He applied the strategy of aggregating marginal gains, which consists of seeking the smallest possible improvement (say 1%) in everything we do to achieve a significant increase when they are added up. This is the same principle that governs stock market growth or successful YouTube channels, for example.

Brailsford and his team optimized all the parameters involved in a cycling race and its preparation: the saddles, the tires, the clothing, the massage gels, etc.

The results were not long in coming: between 2007 and 2017, British cyclists won 178 world championships, 66 Olympic or Paralympic gold medals, and 5 victories in the Tour de France. This illustrates the interest and importance of making small improvements continuously in the long term. If you gain 1% per day, you get more than 37% cumulative improvement after a year (1.01 to the power of 365 = 37.78).

This strategy allows for a **progressive approach**, especially when initiating a transformation when you are in a state of advanced fatigue or stress. It's ultimately like eating an elephant... you end up getting there bite by bite.

3. The "if... then" strategy

American swimmer **Michael Phelps**, the most decorated Olympic athlete of all time with 33 gold medals in his career, regularly used the "if... then" strategy.

Every evening, in preparation for the races, Phelps imagined positive and negative scenarios (the "if") and mentally trained to react to each of them (the "then").

In addition, his coach, **Bob Bowman**, created challenges for him during training and less important competitions so that he would practice responding to these scenarios. Bowman deliberately stepped on Phelps's swimming goggles before a World Cup race in Australia and cracked them. Phelps didn't notice that his goggles were broken until he dived into the pool, and they suddenly filled with water. He didn't let it affect him. Indeed, Bowman and he had developed a strategy during training to know exactly how many arm strokes it took to swim a length.

Intentionally stepping on Phelps's goggles may seem like a useless exercise, but Bowman believes that athletes must **be prepared to**

face all types of scenarios they might encounter in more important competitions. In other words, if an unexpected event like this happened during a race, remembering to count his arm strokes would help Phelps focus on the fast-swimming process and deal with the situation.

This is exactly what happened during one of Phelps's biggest races, the final of the 200-meter butterfly at the 2008 Olympic Games. In the middle of the race, Phelps's goggles started to fill with water. He could no longer see the lane markers at the bottom of the pool, the wall at the end of the pool, or even his competitors. He was suddenly swimming in the dark.

Rather than panicking, Phelps remained calm. As he had done in Australia, he began counting his arm strokes in the last lap, knowing it would take him 21 strokes to swim a length. He increased his pace halfway and approached the wall after the 21st arm stroke, resulting in a new gold medal and a world record.

Exercise: The table below provides a structure for the exercise. Start by listing each "if" in the first column. In the second, define a corresponding "then" for how you would like to react. The example given includes various healthy options for responding to a craving for an unhealthy snack.

IF... (opportunity or obstacle)	THEN... (more useful response)
If I feel like eating an unhealthy snack...	I will drink water / I will eat a fruit / I will go for a walk / I will brush my teeth instead.

4. The strategy of happiness

We generally feel happy when our living conditions meet our ideal blueprint. Therefore, we feel unhappy when this is not the case, and even worse, we suffer when we believe we can't do anything about it and feel powerless.

However, we can always either **change** our current living conditions (this book is full of advice on how to do it) or review our ideals (it may happen that we have a false idea of what we really want), or act on both.

In his book "The Code of the Extraordinary Mind", **Vishen Lakhiani** explains that it is important to keep in mind 2 key elements to be happy:

- knowing how to **enjoy the present moment** by being grateful for everything we already have

Indeed, we are often richer than we think (in the broadest sense of the term). The beneficial effects of **gratitude** are multiplied when we manage to immerse ourselves again in the pleasant moments of the past by seeing what we saw, hearing what we heard, and feeling what we felt. Personally, I practice this exercise every morning by recalling 3 past moments for which I am truly grateful. I vary these moments almost every day by reconnecting primarily with the most recent events.

- having a **positive vision of the future**

Feeling progress contributes to happiness, as does thinking that tomorrow will be even better than today. Set goals related to your ideals and make sure they are a mix of easily achievable goals (to get results and maintain motivation) and much more ambitious goals, with a lower likelihood of success but a much more significant impact.

5. The strategy for finding love

If you are currently single, or if you expect more from your current relationship, ask yourself **who you should become** to attract the person you are looking for.

It can be useful to rethink your past stories to identify their repetitive patterns, those that you unconsciously repeat and that no longer serve you. It can be a way of expressing yourself (too direct, too aggressive), of not expressing yourself (unsaid things), or perhaps a lack of self-confidence because you don't like your physique. If so, what can you improve? Lose weight? Change your look? Get orthodontic treatment? There is always something to do to get closer to what you want. Take action!

6. Modeling

"Success leaves clues. Go figure out what someone who was successful did, and model it. Then improve it but learn their steps. They have knowledge." Tony Robbins

When you want to cook a specific dish, you most likely follow a **recipe** that has already proven itself. This is the idea of modeling: observing successful behaviors, determining the conditions for success, and replicating them as best as possible. Modeling is an important branch of NLP, Neuro-Linguistic Programming, in which I am a certified Master Practitioner.

In a simplified version, modeling is fortunately within everyone's reach; you just need to question people around you who have succeeded where you want to.

Another tip is to read **autobiographies** of inspiring people, whether in the field you are interested in (e.g. football) or in a much broader way. I personally like to read several books on different topics in parallel because it allows me to make richer and more innovative mental connections.

Another strategy is to mentally form a kind of **council of wise people** (or board of directors to use a more business term) of real, living, or not, or imaginary personalities, and see what they could advise you on a given issue. One day, I formed one with **Tony Robbins, Gandhi, James Bond** (personalized by **Daniel Craig**), and **Gandalf**. The messages received were: "take more action", "be patient, big changes take time", "dress better", and "stay true to your values and your code of honor even if it won't always be easy". Do the exercise, you might be surprised by what emerges.

You can also obviously model yourself by comparing how you behave in a successful situation versus a failure situation. For example, how do you make your decisions in one situation and in the other? Certainly not in the same way!

STRATEGIES OF FAILURE

There are also strategies of failure that we all unconsciously repeat, to procrastinate or even to be sad or depressed for example. These strategies prevent us from giving our best. They define our **upper limit** and therefore have a negative impact on the results we obtain.

I present to you 4 general ones below:

1. Judging or criticizing

This is probably the most important failure strategy: judging or criticizing others, external conditions, or yourself (or all three). It often comes into play when you don't feel happy, that is, when your current living conditions are not aligned with your ideal. It will be much more profitable to **take responsibility** and take action where you can and let go where you cannot act.

Our **inner judge** is our greatest saboteur, especially since we are rarely fully aware of its existence and importance. In his book "Positive Intelligence", **Shirzad Chamine** describes 9 accomplice saboteurs:

- the Avoider,
- the Controller,
- the Hyper-Achiever,
- the Hyper-Rational,
- the Hyper-Vigilant,
- the Pleaser,
- the Restless,
- the Stickler and
- the Victim.

These saboteurs are universal because they are connected to areas of our brain linked to our survival. We develop them in early childhood to survive the physical and emotional threats we perceive at that time, through our child's eyes. They are no longer useful to us as adults, although they remain present without our knowledge.

You can identify the most important ones for you on the website https://www.positiveintelligence.com/saboteurs.

2. Taking failures personally

Your perception of what failure is can affect your self-confidence and slow you down in your development. Instead, see each "failure" as a **learning experience** and as a step that brings you even closer to your goal by enriching your deliberate practice (see below).

3. Getting stuck and inactive when something goes wrong

Keep in mind the 3 states of self-mastery: how you feel, how you think, and how you act. If you feel stuck, it is very likely that you are oscillating between 2 of these states, let's say your thoughts and your emotions. Then move to the third, action in the given example. When I am struggling with strong negative emotions, going around in my head, and not having much energy to train, I do my ironing. This action allows me to change states in 30 to 45 minutes (and then have the satisfaction of the work done).

If you don't get the expected results, stay in motion and keep testing. Life is like an escalator; you have to step on it for it to start moving.

4. **Refusing compliments or gifts that come your way**

To be in abundance and progress, there is nothing worse than refusing what comes to you. Accept what is offered to you and reciprocate by thanking the person for the gift they have given you.

HABITS

"We are what we repeatedly do. Excellence, therefore, is not an act, but a habit." Aristotle

Whatever your dreams or the principles and strategies you wish to apply, they will only materialize if you establish the corresponding habits. By habit, I mean a behavior that has been repeated enough to become **automatic**.

Unfortunately, the system in which we live does not teach us the essentials, let alone how to function at our best.

The good news is that it is up to you to reverse the trend and establish better habits day after day, week after week, month after month, year after year.

I would like to share with you the story of **Steve Martin**, a famous American actor, comedian, musician, and screenwriter.

At around 10 years old, he started selling books at Disneyland, which had just opened its doors in California. Within a year, he moved to the magic workshop, where he learned tricks from older employees. He experimented with jokes and tried simple routines on visitors. Soon, he discovered that he enjoyed performing and set his mind on becoming a comedian.

From adolescence, he performed in small clubs in Los Angeles. His show was short, and he rarely stayed on stage for more than five minutes. The crowds were small, and most of the audience didn't even pay attention to him. One night, he literally performed his stand-up routine in an empty club. Nevertheless, he gradually extended his stage time, and his skills continued to develop.

At nineteen, he performed every week for twenty minutes. He spent another ten years experimenting, adapting, and training. He then accepted a job as a writer for television and gradually managed to make his own appearances on talk shows. In the mid-1970s, he became a regular guest on "The Tonight Show" and "Saturday Night Live", two iconic shows in the United States.

Finally, after nearly fifteen years of work, Steve Martin achieved fame. He toured sixty cities in sixty-three days, then seventy-two cities in eighty days, and then eighty-five cities in ninety days. At a show in Ohio, 18,695 people attended the performance. Another 45,000 tickets were sold for his three-day show in New York. He was propelled to the pinnacle of his art and became one of the most popular comedians of his time.

His story provides a fascinating perspective on what it takes to stick to your habits in the long term. To quote his words, "ten years of learning, four years of perfecting, and four years of crazy success."

What is fantastic is that our habits are somewhat like **mobile applications**; we can delete them, update them, or even download new ones.

If you want to improve your life, you must improve your habits... constantly. This brings us back to the notion of **training and path**. This is how you will gradually and exponentially gain efficiency and productivity in the areas that truly matter to you. To save time, you can obviously draw inspiration from the habits of successful people, especially if they have already achieved what you want to accomplish.

Here are some important points to help you:

- switch to **discovery** mode

It's a bit like exploring the app store on your smartphone or tablet. You might discover one that you hadn't thought of but that will be particularly useful to you.

- **refresh** your habits regularly

Update your 'applications,' for example, once a month, quarter, or year.

- establish a system to **measure** the effectiveness of your habits

You will thus know which ones are the most effective and/or best suited to you.

- be clear about your **limits**

For example, what is the maximum weight you are willing to reach? How many consecutive days without exercise do you want to tolerate?

- **adjust** what needs to be based on the results obtained and your living conditions

You can, for example, accept to lower certain criteria if you have to deal with more challenges or workload temporarily. Even the Formula 1 World Champion does not constantly drive at maximum speed. Adaptation is crucial!

But how do you actually establish a better habit? According to **James Clear**, it involves using a 4-step model: the cue, craving, response, and reward.

- **the cue**

This is what **stimulates** your nervous system to initiate a behavior in order to obtain a reward (for our ancestors, mainly water, food, or sex; for us today, money, fame, social status, congratulations, approval, love and friendship, or personal satisfaction).

- **the craving**

This is the motivation behind every habit. Without **motivation** or desire, you have no reason to act. Cravings differ from person to person and are not triggered by the same signals for everyone. As seen earlier, self-discipline also comes into play at this stage.

- **the response**

This is the **habit itself,** which can take the form of a thought or an action. The response only occurs if you are motivated enough and if you encounter little friction. The response also depends on your skills (see below).

- **the reward**

This is the ultimate goal of each habit, **satisfying** your cravings and teaching you what works best.

To establish a **new habit**, it is ideal to act simultaneously on each of these steps, by making the action both:

- **obvious** (to favor the trigger),
- **attractive** (to create desire),
- **easy** to accomplish (to provide a result), and
- **enjoyable** (to encourage repetition).

Conversely, to get rid of a **bad habit,** you will need to make it both:

- as **invisible** as possible (to avoid the trigger),
- **unattractive** (to decrease the craving),
- **difficult** (to interfere with the response), and
- **unpleasant** (so that there is no reward).

According to various authors, the duration of establishing a new habit takes an average of 66 days (between 18 and 254 days) depending on the habit being established. It can therefore be very quick.

Keep in mind that a little is better than nothing, and opt for **progressiveness**. Therefore, make sure that your new habit does not take more than 2 minutes at the beginning so that it is very easy to establish. For example, "reading before bed" will initially be "reading one page". You can then increase the duration.

I will conclude this section with 3 tips that will guarantee the

establishment of new habits:
- **stack** them on other existing habits,
- **adapt** them to your environment (and vice versa),
- follow and **measure** them.

Exercise: Examine your current habits and identify areas where you can improve. Then establish clear goals and concrete action plans to achieve them.

SKILLS

No matter what habits we put in place to achieve our dreams, they will only be effective if we are competent in their implementation.

According to **Robert B. Dilts** & **Mickey A. Feher**, our skills are generally evaluated based on 3 dimensions:

- whether we enjoy doing the action or not,
- whether we do it well and
- whether we spend time on it.

If you tick all three boxes, and your actions are in line with your passion, mission, and ambition, then you are in your **zone of genius.**

If you tick all three boxes, but your actions are not entirely in line with your passion, mission, and ambition, then you are in your **zone of excellence.**

If you enjoy the activity and do it well but do not spend time on it, you are in an **unexploited zone of excellence.**

If you do the activity well and spend time on it but do not enjoy it, you are in your **competence zone.**

If you are good at something, don't enjoy doing it, and don't spend time on it, you are in an **unexploited competence zone.**

If you enjoy the activity, spend time on it, but are not particularly good at it, it is more like a **hobby.**

If you enjoy the activity but are not particularly good at it and don't dedicate much time to it, it is an **interest.**

If you spend time doing something you neither enjoy nor do well, you are in the **incompetence zone.**

If you don't check any of the boxes, the activity will be a **waste of time** for you.

Keep in mind that these 3 dimensions are **interconnected**; the more you enjoy something, the more likely you are to spend time on it and become good at it (if you apply deliberate practice). And the more time you spend and become good at it, the more you will probably enjoy it. Therefore, it can be useful to train to become better and plan practice time to progress (consistency before quantity).

We experience maximum motivation when we work on tasks that are at the limits of our current abilities. Not too difficult. Not too easy. Just right.

LEARNING

"Do the best you can until you know better. Then, when you know better, do better." Maya Angelou

The development of your skills inevitably goes through learning. And what would be the first thing to learn, in your opinion? Well, it is how to **learn to learn**!

Speed reading techniques, **mind mapping**, and **memorization** should be taught first in school. Since this is not yet the case (everywhere), it is up to you to discover them for yourself and share them with your children.

To whet your appetite and inspire you to delve deeper into these subjects, I will share two tips among the many that exist.

To **read faster**, simply use your finger or a pen and follow the text, accelerating compared to reading without support. A young teenager of 12 years old whom I recently supported increased his reading speed by 50%! Imagine the time saved for his homework, tests, and his entire school career! Not to mention that reading faster requires the brain to be more active, a bit like when you drive a car; the faster you go, the more focused you are. Obviously, there is a speed beyond which it becomes ineffective (and dangerous in the example of driving a car).

Another tip is to **use colors** when using mind mapping; this will also activate your brain more and thus your cognitive abilities.

DELIBERATE PRACTICE

The discovery of deliberate practice was a real revelation for me. The best illustration I know of is the story of Top Gun, the United States Navy Fighter Weapons School popularized by the movie of the same name starring **Tom Cruise**.

During the Vietnam War, the performance of American pilots had dropped to 1 enemy aircraft shot down for every 1 American aircraft, which was not very cost-effective, neither in terms of human lives nor financially (given the cost of a fighter jet). The Americans then implemented deliberate practice, resulting in a ratio of 12 enemy aircraft shot down for every American aircraft between 1970 and 1973. During the 7 months of the first Gulf War, American pilots shot down 33 enemy aircraft in aerial combat, losing only one aircraft during the operation, making it probably the most striking performance in the history of aerial combat.

But what does this famous deliberate practice consist of, you may ask? First, it involves selecting **recognized experts** in their field (here, seasoned veteran pilots) and putting the apprentices (who have also undergone a selection process) in conditions as close as possible to the **reality** of the field. Then, each practical session is followed by a **debriefing** that highlights the behaviors that worked well and those that need to be improved. Gradually, the students gain both competence and confidence. This is very well illustrated in the movie.

Deliberate practice is the **key to the success** of World Champions in various fields such as chess, music, and sports.

The number of hours of practice, in other words, training, is obviously important, but it is above all the quality of it that will make the difference. Surround yourself with competent people and gradually implement positive behaviors while getting rid of those that do not serve you. In a short time, and in line with the strategy of marginal gains, you will be surprised by the results you will achieve.

TOOLS

I present in this section some tools that will be useful to you and deserve to be used regularly.

In a couple or group performance context (whether in sports or in a professional setting), this will help you to know yourself better. Then, share the individual results and capitalize on complementarities.

The identity matrix

How can you effectively embark on a personal development journey without knowing yourself? This is the goal of the identity matrix, which allows you to discover yourself along three axes: **who you are, who you can become,** and **who you are not.** Each of these is then divided into **who you want to be** and **who you do not want to be.**

It is important to understand that the matrix thus highlights the **beliefs** you have about yourself rather than absolute truths. Therefore, **everything is possible** in terms of change and evolution.

The table below presents the different elements in a more visual manner.

	I am	I could become	I am not
I want to be	Your center (pride, satisfaction)	Your potential (hope, excitement)	Your limits (frustration, sorrow)
I don't want to be	Your shadows (shame, guilt)	Vos flaws ou weaknesses (fear, anxiety)	Your frontiers (freedom)

Values and code of honor

We have seen earlier the importance of **needs** and **value**s in satisfying them in the way that best suits us. By having a clear vision of your values, you will have a code of honor similar to the samurai who followed Bushido.

I suggest you do the exercise by reflecting on both **your current situation** and **the one you want to achieve**. For each of these columns, list in order of importance the values that **attract** you (those to which you associate **pleasure**) and those you want to **avoid** (because you associate **suffering** with them), your anti-values in a way.

Make sure not to list one of the six needs as a "value" (such as love, for example) to avoid any redundancy. We all have the 6 needs, not necessarily in the same order, but not the same values.

In the example presented, the value "sincerity" has increased in priority in the desired state column. This can be useful if you want to increase the quality of your relationships, for example.

The value "curiosity" has been added in the desired state column. It will be beneficial if you are regularly confronted with the same problem for which you cannot find a solution. Being more curious will help you open up possibilities and have a more open mind.

Values corresponding to your current state		Values corresponding to your desired state	
Attractive values	Repulsive values	Attractive values	Repulsive values
Integrity	Disrespect	Integrity	Injustice
Courage	Injustice	Sincerity	Disrespect
Learning	Betrayal	Curiosity	Betrayal
Sincerity	/	Learning	/

Once your values are identified, think about what you need for them to be experienced and felt. Most people consider themselves to have the value of respect but may express it in very different ways. The same goes for freedom.

In a couple or an organization, identifying common values is not enough; you must agree on a **clear and common definition** of these values. Otherwise, it may create confusion and tension.

Strength profile

To achieve the set goals, certain qualities or strengths will be more important, or even crucial, than others. They may vary depending on the stage you are at (hence the importance of revisiting the exercise regularly).

Having a clear vision (we come back to the importance of clarity) is therefore key for you. List the **required qualities**, evaluate your current score for each of them, the desired score, and how you will bridge the gap (if there is one).

The table below gives you an example, with three strengths, two of which require an action plan.

Be as **specific** as possible in defining the **action** and make sure to progress gradually (see the section on habits).

Strength	Current level	Desired level	How to work on it
Serenity	7	9	5 minutes of heart coherence per day
Concentration	5	8	Implement the Pomodoro technique
Motivation	9	9	/

Focus and concentration

Two techniques are conducive to focus and concentration.

The first is to get into a state of **flow** (also known as "being in the zone"). For this, your goals must be clear, you must be able to have immediate feedback on your progress, and your challenges must be tailored to your skills, perhaps slightly above.

The second is to get into the state of **engagement** where you ensure that what needs to happen happens (without thinking). It will be very useful when your performance goals are set, and the situation is physically and/or mentally exhausting.

It is also important to distinguish between what we can control and what we cannot, and to focus only on the former.

You can thus establish pre-performance routines (preparation of equipment, visualization, etc.) and post-performance routines (for example, taking 10 steps after throwing the basketball, even if the shot is bad).

Controllable	Uncontrollable
My mental state	The behavior of the audience
My focus & my concentration	The importance of the match
My physical engagement	The competition venue
My schedule	Weather conditions

You can also work on your internal dialogue by using **triggering words** or phrases, such as technical ones ("move, position, strike") or behavioral ones ("calm, confidence, and control"). You can also be more directive and silence it when it is not useful to you ("shut up!").
Take time to explore the modalities of your "inner voice". You will be surprised by the effects you can achieve with a few small changes.

Priming

The goal of priming is to best **prepare you** for what is to come. It can be your day, your evening, an important meeting, a writing session, a fitness session, an intimate moment with someone, and so on.

It is a strategy that I personally use every day.

Priming must consider two points: **your current state** and **your desired state**. If you are tired or exhausted and need to perform, your priming should boost you. Conversely, if you are excited and need to rest and recover, your priming should promote relaxation.

Priming acts on both your physiology/biochemistry and your psychology.

The priming of your **body** is generally known as warm-up. It prepares your muscles, tendons, cardiovascular system, and nervous system for performance.

Priming has also been studied for years in **psychology**. It can have a significant impact on your behavior and habits, often without you realizing it. Priming related to preliminaries occurs because you store information in your long-term memory in the form of groups, or "schemas". For example, when you see a word or an image, the rest of the group to which it belongs is also activated, and the corresponding information is easier to obtain.

In a study conducted in 2008 by psychologists at Yale, participants were asked to hold their coffee for 10 to 25 seconds in the elevator that took them to the laboratory. The researcher then noted some information about the participant before asking them to return their coffee. For half of the participants, the coffee was hot, while for the other half, it was cold. That was the only difference between the two groups of participants. Here is where things get interesting. In the laboratory, all participants read the same brief description of a randomly chosen person and evaluated their personality using a questionnaire. Participants holding the hot coffee judged the person to be happier, more natural, more generous, and more social. Participants holding the cold cup were more likely to say that the person was unhappy, irritable, and selfish. Remember that there was absolutely no difference between the profiles read by the two groups. However, the way they reacted to the descriptions was very different depending on how they were "primed".

You have also undoubtedly experienced the phenomenon of **emotional priming**. Think of a time when you were angry or frustrated; did you then overreact to a small problem? Did the situation seem worse because you were still clinging to the event that made you angry? Well, that is because you had felt the priming effect of your anger, which then prompted you to react that way.

Now think of a time when you were completely happy or in love, for example. Did everything seem easier to handle? That is because you had been primed with a pleasant feeling.

You will also find an example of priming in the movie "Focus" with **Will Smith** and **Margot Robbie** during the scene with the choice of the American football player's number.

Your thoughts, feelings, and emotions can be stimulated by factors of which you are not even aware, with a considerable impact on your performance in other aspects of your life. Practiced regularly, priming will help you cultivate positive emotions and significantly improve your quality of life.

Several priming techniques can be used, ideally in combination. Here are 6 important ones.

- **Music** is probably the easiest way to change your state. Identify songs that impact your mood or even create playlists that can be used whenever needed (for example, handpans for yoga or concentration, etc.).

- The **respiratory system** is the only system capable of functioning autonomously and controlled. Inhalation is related to the branch of the autonomic nervous system (called sympathetic) while exhalation is rather related to the relaxation branch (parasympathetic). So, if you want to stimulate yourself, use a longer tempo for inhalation and a shorter one for exhalation. For example, start by exhaling deeply, then inhale deeply for 4 seconds and exhale for 1 second. If you want to relax, do the opposite; for example, inhale for 4 seconds by inflating your belly (especially on the sides as most gas exchanges occur in the lower part of the lungs) and exhale for 8 seconds by contracting it. Repeat the process for a few minutes until you feel a difference in your state.

- Another tip to improve mental clarity is to increase your oxygen intake by doing some **powerful breathing**, ideally outside, or at least where the air is quite fresh (avoid toilets).

There are many other breathing techniques, such as heart coherence (inhale for 5 seconds, exhale for 5 seconds, repeat for 5 minutes, 3 times a day). Feel free to try some and choose the one that suits you best.

- The practice of **mindfulness** combines very well with breathing. It involves focusing on the present moment in a non-judgmental way by focusing on our sensory perceptions (sight, hearing, sensations, etc.). It is also a very good exercise to decrease the impact of our saboteurs (see above) and gradually decrease their neural connections.

- **Imagination**, often (in my opinion, wrongly) called visualization, consists of mentally creating a dynamic or relaxing environment. Think, for example, of an athlete in competition or a view of the ocean, respectively. Include details such as colors, an enlarged or reduced view, depending on what suits you best (we are not all equal in this respect).

- In her famous 2012 TED talk, **Amy Cuddy** explains that a change in posture can affect your physiology and therefore your state in just 2 minutes. In short, power poses (think of Spiderman or Wonder Woman) can increase your testosterone and decrease your cortisol, and thereby boost your confidence level. Conversely, a low-power pose will lead to a lack of confidence, etc. Her study has been refuted by other psychologists, but I personally use it and feel the beneficial effects. Try it out and form your own opinion.

Want to energize yourself quickly? Try some jumping jacks or any other movement suitable for your attire. Need to gain serenity? Do a few yoga poses.

You can increase the effects and speed of action of these various points by **combining** them. Other factors such as exposure to the sun, specific smells (e.g. essential oils), earthing or grounding (direct contact with the Earth), singing, or even trampolining can also be beneficial.

Routines

As we have seen previously, we achieve results in line with what we do regularly. Routines will, therefore, be very important, especially those in the morning and in the evening.

It is obviously not always possible to dedicate an hour each day to this, although the results obtained will depend on the quality time you allocate to them. Define both your **optimal routine** (to be done, for example, on weekends) and your **minimal routine** that you will do no matter what, even if you are traveling, for example.

For the morning routine, your goal will be to energize yourself and prepare for a day of quality in terms of joy and productivity. As for me, my morning routine at the time of writing this book is as follows:

- I wake up,
- I rinse my mouth (to eliminate waste generated during the night and to avoid putting extra burden on my body for cleaning) and my face,
- I may go back to bed to perform some Osteostrong mobility exercises,
- I go down and hang for about thirty seconds on a pull-up bar to take care of my spine and maintain sufficient extension,

- I continue with Osteostrong exercises and include around 150 sit-ups,
- I do **Tony Robbins'** priming, which includes, among other things, the gratitude exercise and goal visualization (this is also my minimal routine; whatever happens, I do at least the priming) and
- I have breakfast.

You can also add a cold shower, reading, learning, and/or work on a personal project that is dear to you.

For the evening routine, the goal will be relaxation and preparation for a night and quality rest. You can include reading (with a real book, especially to avoid screens), gentle stretching, and a hot bath. Intimate moments are also welcome (especially if you are in a relationship).

Anchors and symbols

The term "anchoring" refers to the process of associating an internal response with an environmental or mental trigger to quickly elicit a desired response. It is a technique widely used in NLP (Neuro-Linguistic Programming).

This process is very similar to the conditioning technique used by **Ivan Pavlov**, the famous Russian physiologist and Nobel laureate in Physiology or Medicine in 1904. By associating the sound of a bell with feeding dogs, he discovered that he could trigger the dogs' salivation merely by ringing the bell, even if no food was provided.

The anchoring **process** can be used to help you remember and activate your internal resources when you need them. For instance, by associating a gesture, a sound, or an image (or all three) with a state (let's say relaxation), you can quickly experience this state just by triggering the chosen gesture, sound, and/or image. Anchors can be stacked to achieve combined and amplified effects.

Objects or symbols can also serve as your anchors. I have a habit of collecting mugs from the countries I have the pleasure of visiting. In September 2023, I discovered Iceland, which was no exception. I brought back a beautiful mug featuring the symbol Ægishjálmur for protection and invincibility in battle. I enjoy using this mug in challenging moments when I feel the need to boost my inner strength.

Former President **Barack Obama** also always carries a few small objects with him. These are mementos gathered from his encounters that hold special meaning for him, such as a rosary gifted by Pope Francis, a small Buddha received from a Buddhist monk, a small statue of the Hindu monkey god Hanuman given by a woman, and a Coptic cross from Ethiopia.

When he feels tired or discouraged, he simply rummages through his pocket and thinks to himself, "Yes, I can overcome this because people have entrusted me with the privilege of working on these issues that directly affect them".

How about you? Do you harness the power of symbols? If something is currently missing for you, what symbol could represent it?

Action plan

To progress from your current situation to your desired state, define an action plan as concretely as possible, and review it regularly (for example, once a week) to track your progress and update it. Below is a suggested format, but feel free to adapt it to best suit your needs.

ACTION	TARGET	DEADLINE	STATUS
Write a book	Minimum 100 pages	31/10/2023	In progress
Yoga	3 times/week	None	/
Purchase an earthing mat	/	15/09/2023	Done

RISKS

Tackling ambitious goals, perhaps never previously achieved, at least by you, carries risks.

A risk is defined as the **likelihood** of a problem occurring multiplied by the **impact** it will have if it does. The human mind (perhaps this is indeed a cognitive bias?) tends to attach more importance to the likelihood ("this won't happen to me") rather than the impact.

In Belgium, and in other European countries, we experienced a wave of floods in 2021, some of which caused (more or less directly) a tsunami-like rise in water to the first floor of certain houses. The probability of such an event was extremely low, but the impact was dramatic.

In the pursuit of ambitious goals, it will be much more useful to seek a **favorable asymmetry**, as explained by **Nassim Nicholas**

Taleb in his book "Antifragile: things that gain from disorder". In short, the idea is to have much more to gain than to lose in case of difficulties, meaning that the probability of losing can be high if the impact is low. Conversely, we will not shy away from actions that have a low probability of success but an enormous impact if success is achieved.

CHALLENGES

"Problems call us to a higher level." Tony Robbins

It inevitably happens that we encounter challenges, **difficult moments**. The worst are those that last a long time and accumulate.

In those moments, all the tools presented in this book will be useful to you, and it might even be a good time to reread it.

I would like to emphasize three essential aspects for your resilience in particular:

- reconnect with your **positive vision** of the future

If necessary, improve it. Convince yourself that tomorrow will be better than today.

- find **people** to support and guide you

If you don't have such people in your immediate circle, it may be time to turn to a coach. If you don't have that option, create one. Besides saving time with valuable advice, not feeling alone will be of great help to you.

- take **action**

Test, explore, create opportunities for yourself. Adjust your plan, if necessary, but keep moving.

Challenges are often transitional moments aimed at taking us to the next level. Simply seeing them that way will already be more beneficial for you. When this happens to me, I often think of **Abraham Lincoln**, who is probably one of the best examples of motivation and **perseverance** one can find. His life was initially a succession of misfortunes and failures.

1816: The Lincolns are forced out of their home. At the age of 7, Abraham has to work to support the family.

1818: Death of his mother

1831: First bankruptcy

1832: Beaten in the legislative elections

1832: Loses his job and is rejected for admission to law school

1833: Borrows money from a friend to start a business and goes bankrupt before the end of the year (he spends 17 years of his life repaying this debt)

1834: Elected to the legislative elections

1835: Death of his fiancée

1836: Severe nervous breakdown (bedridden for six months)

1838: Beaten for the Presidency of the Illinois House of

Representatives

1846: Elected to Congress and goes to Washington where he does good work

1848: Not re-elected for a second term in Congress

1849: Applies for the job of land agent in his home state and does not get it

1854: Beaten when he runs for the United States Senate

1856: Gets fewer than a hundred votes when he runs for the vice presidency at the national party convention

1858: Beaten when he runs for the Senate again

1860: Elected President of the United States

1864: Re-elected in 1864

He could have given up several times, but he did not. And because he never gave up, he became **one of the greatest** presidents of the United States by abolishing slavery in 1865, before being assassinated a few months later.

One could argue that all his challenges actually prepared and toughened him to be able to lead a torn country to more humanity, which perhaps no one else could have done. So, stay the course during the storm and have faith in your final destination.

FAILURES

"Failure is success in progress." Albert Einstein

Failure is part of the process. Yet, it is probably the most difficult to handle, especially in the long run.

Even in school, the red annotations from the teacher negatively stimulate us. And as long as our parents do not have the required maturity (I am convinced that there should be a license or at least training before becoming a parent), they pile on when we get home.

Failure also has a **cultural dimension**; in the United States, for example, failing to launch an entrepreneurial project is much more valued than in Europe. In Silicon Valley, there is an entrepreneur mantra that says, "Fail fast, learn fast". It even seems that those who failed early, and learned from it, will succeed better and faster than those who had a smooth journey.

The more you take action, the more you will fail, especially in the beginning, and the more you will succeed later. This is what **Michael Jordan** tells us: "I have missed more than 9,000 shots in my career. I have lost almost 300 games. 26 times, I have been trusted to take the game-winning shot and missed. I have failed over and over and over again in my life. And that is why I succeed."

In his book "Les vertus de l'échec", **Charles Pepin** notably discusses how failure can help us better understand, learn faster, explore, open new paths, strengthen our character, build humility, experience real life, and reinvent ourselves.

Always remember that failure is a learning experience... only if you know how to leverage it through **deliberate practice** described earlier.

Finally, **ignore negative people**, especially on social media where they are increasingly present, and stay focused on your goals. If necessary, evolve your circle by surrounding yourself with people with a growth mindset.

FOR MORE INFORMATION

Abraham Lincoln, https://en.wikipedia.org/wiki/Abraham_Lincoln

Antifragile: Things That Gain from Disorder, Nassim Nicholas Taleb, 2014

Atomic Habits: An Easy & Proven Way to Build Good Habits & Break Bad Ones, James Clear, 2018

Awaken the Giant Within: How to Take Immediate Control of Your Mental, Emotional, Physical & Financial Destiny, Anthony Robbins, 1991

Giant Steps: Small Changes to Make a Big Difference, Tony Robbins, 1994

Hanuman's Figurine Is President Barack Obama's Lucky Charm, 2016, https://economictimes.indiatimes.com/news/politics-and-nation/hanuman-figurine-is-president-barack-obamas-lucky-charm/articleshow/50603496.cms

How Should I Start Each Day? What Is Priming? https://www.tonyrobbins.com/ask-tony/priming

L'Effet Placebo En Toute Transparence, Kheira Bettayeb, 2023, https://lejournal.cnrs.fr/articles/leffet-placebo-en-toute-transparence

Les Vertus de l'Echec, Charles Pépin, 2018

Mind Map Mastery: The Complete Guide to Learning and Using the Most Powerful Thinking Tool in The Universe, Tony Buzan, 2018

Mind Set Win S2 E1, F1 Champion Max Verstappen On Trusting The Process, https://www.redbull.com/int-en/podcast-episodes/mind-set-win-s2-e1-max-verstappen

Modeling with NLP, Robert Dilts, 1998

Peak: How All of Us Can Achieve Extraordinary Things, Anders Ericsson & Robert Pool, 2017

Positive Intelligence: Why Only 20% Of Teams And Individuals Achieve Their True Potential And How You Can Achieve Yours, Shirzad Chamine, 2012

Power Posing Is Back: Amy Cuddy Successfully Refutes Criticism, Kim Elsesser, 2018, https://www.forbes.com/sites/kimelsesser/2018/04/03/power-posing-is-back-amy-cuddy-successfully-refutes-criticism/?sh=686dd79d3b8e

Pressing Reset: Original Strength Reloaded, Tim Anderson & Geoff Neupert, 2017

Success Factor Modeling Volumes I-III, Robert Brian Dilts and Antonio Meza, 2015-2017

The Big Leap: Conquer Your Hidden Fear and Take Life to The Next Level, Gay Hendricks, 2010

The Code of the Extraordinary Mind: 10 Unconventional Laws to Redefine Your Life and Succeed on Your Own Terms, Vishen Lakhiani, 2016

The Genius of Athletes: What World-Class Competitors Know That Can Change Your Life, Noel Brick & Scott Douglas, 2021

The Power of Mindset Change: Why Mindset Matters Most, Robert B Dilts & Mickey Feher, 2023

Unlimited Power, Anthony Robbins, 1986

Un Optimiste Persévérant : Abraham Lincoln, https://www.liguedesoptimistes.fr/2012/10/28/un-optimiste-perseverant-abraham-lincoln

Your Body Language May Shape Who You Are, Amy Cuddy, 2012, TED talk, https://www.ted.com/talks/amy_cuddy_your_body_languag-may_shape_who_you_are/transcript

5 - LET GO

"Train yourself to let go of everything you fear to lose." Master Yoda

"Do nothing that is of no use." Myamoto Musashi

"If you resist change, you resist life." Sadhguru

"Tension is who you think you should be, relaxation is who you are."
Chinese proverb

We have previously seen the many benefits of self-mastery. However, there are situations where things do not go as planned, both in business and in love, for example, especially when other **people** are involved. You may feel frustration, stress, or even anger.

If you **resist** what is happening, desperately trying to maintain control over everything, you will **exhaust** yourself unnecessarily.

At some point, you must realize that some things may be beyond your control, that life can be unpredictable and chaotic, that failures and setbacks are an integral part of your life, and that some people do not deserve you. It is then time to let go. Instead of resisting, learn to **adapt and grow** through these experiences.

QUITE AN ART

Letting go is first about **releasing** everything that no longer serves you (thoughts, beliefs, habits, etc.). If you feel weighed down, lighten your load!

This could be the right time for a **detox**, whether it is through dietary changes, to purify your liver and promote internal hygiene, or in your relationships, to decrease certain negative influences. It could also be an opportune moment for a digital break from social media, reducing unnecessary nerve stimulation (especially towards the end of the day). Letting go will give you a breath of fresh air that will do you a world of good (consider reconnecting with nature, particularly the marine or forest environment).

Letting go may also require **unlearning** through self-reflection and the development of a more critical thinking.

Often, our stress stems from unrealistic expectations or fear of change. Learn to **manage your expectations** by being realistic about what you can control. Accept that life has its ups and downs, and not everything will always go as planned.

Perfectionism can also be a significant source of stress. Accept that you don't have to be perfect and be kind to yourself and others.

Make a list of your tasks and concerns. Identify what is truly important and what can wait. **Focus** on the **priority** items and let go of what is not essential. This will help lighten your mental load. Successful people have learned to say "no" much more frequently to focus more on the essential and on what helps them achieve the desired results.

Letting go is also about trusting what you have already defined and put in place (strategy, routines, team, etc.). Triple Formula 1 World Champion **Max Verstappen** explains it well: "I love what I do, but I don't overthink it - I don't ask myself too many questions. I just go with the flow, and it works for me". Of course, this implies that what has been put in place beforehand has been optimized and is trustworthy.

Letting go is also about savoring what you already have and not necessarily always wanting more (see the happiness strategy in chapter 4 above). Keep a **gratitude** journal. Each day, write down at least three things you are grateful for. This will help focus your mind on the positive.

Letting go is also about knowing how to ask and how to receive. Do you have the habit of praying? If so, silently or out loud? Try both versions, and you will see that it is more powerful out loud. If not, why not? And what if you tried?

To practice letting go, take a moment to sit quietly, close your eyes, take a deep breath in, and exhale slowly. As you release your breath, imagine letting go of all your worries and tensions. Use visualization to symbolically release your worries. See them dissolve or fly away, which will help you mentally let go of your concerns.

Be aware of the present moment without judgment. You can also **meditate** by focusing on a word, an image, or your breath. When thoughts arise, observe them without judgment or attachment, then bring your attention back to your breath, the sounds you hear, the objects around you, or the sensations of what you touch.

Regular meditation and **mindfulness** will help you develop a calmer mind and let go of intrusive thoughts and unnecessary concerns.

TRAPPED EMOTIONS

I have already discussed emotions in this book as they play a crucial role in how we feel and thus in our quality of life.

Letting go can also mean **freeing ourselves** from emotions, whether they are self-generated or absorbed from someone else, for example, from our mother during pregnancy.

From a physical point of view, an emotion is an **electromagnetic current** that seeks to pass through you from bottom to top. If this current stops along the way, thus not passing through you completely, there is stagnant energy, like being trapped and locked in a certain area of your body. It will then create a symptom, more or less significant (pain, dysfunction, and ultimately illness). This is the idea of the famous **"what is not expressed is impressed"**.

When you experience another situation that generates the same sensation, a new wave of energy will pass through you and take with it everything that corresponds to its vibration, gradually rising until it eventually exits the body. The emotion is then fully experienced. Otherwise, the phenomenon will repeat until the emotion can be fully felt.

These trapped emotions can exact a heavy mental and emotional toll, influencing your thought processes, the choices you make, and the level of success and abundance you are able to achieve. Perhaps most damaging of all, trapped emotional energies can accumulate around your **heart**, cutting off your ability to give and receive love.

An average person would have more than a hundred trapped emotions, often without being aware of them. If you have experienced relationship problems, rejection, negative self-talk, loss, or long-term stress, it is highly likely that you have trapped emotions.

The reason why some emotions remain trapped is still not fully understood. It appears that the more overwhelming an emotion is, the higher the likelihood that it remains trapped. There could also be other reasons such as physical weakness or the presence of other similar, older trapped emotions.

Once you have located a trapped emotion, the next step is to **release** it. To do this, an equal and opposite wave of energy must collide with it so that it can be leveled and carried away. This is the same principle as that of noise-canceling headphones, which detect the frequency of external sound waves and produce the opposite frequency to level them.

Living your emotions well is therefore crucial for a good quality of life, good health, and good performance.

Among the useful approaches, we find everything related to vibrations such as **sound therapy** and **shaking** (some animals, like dogs, naturally shake to release their stress). You can also consider energy healing or **magnetism** (as emotions are electromagnetic waves).

I would also add cold baths. I remember discovering **Wim Hof's** method with one of his instructors, **Bart Scholtissen**, shortly after being dismissed in what I considered abusive conditions. Well, I couldn't stop trembling in the icy water, which did not happen again in subsequent baths. I think my body and subconscious thus eliminated a good part of the emotional toxicity I had accumulated during the year leading up to that dismissal.

PRIMITIVES REFLEXES

Can one truly have self-mastery without taking care of one's **body**? I don't think so. This is also true in my opinion when it comes to letting go.

This also involves your primitive reflexes. These are specific **automatic and involuntary reactions** that are triggered by external stimulation (touch, noise, light, etc.). They are necessary for our development (roles of **survival** and **protection**) during which they are supposed to emerge and then integrate, that is, deactivate. If this is not the case, it will most likely result in motor, emotional, and cognitive disturbances. These reflexes can also be reactivated in cases of intense stress, traumatic shock, or illnesses (stroke, Parkinson's, etc.). At least 26 of these reflexes have been identified (Belly Button Radiation, Moro, Galant, Perez, etc.).

If you have difficulty controlling your body during certain **stimulations** (for example, when your feet or belly button are touched) or if you have learning difficulties, consider undergoing an assessment and, if necessary, reintegrating, primarily through movement as described by **Tim Anderson** in his "Original Strength" approach. This is also something I propose in my sessions.

These reflexes are an excellent example of the connections between control and letting go. After all, how can you let go of something that you do not control and that thus controls you?

TOWARDS MORE FREEDOM

Letting go does not mean abandoning your **responsibilities**. On the contrary, it is about freeing your mind from unnecessary burdens and focusing on what is **essential**.

The art of letting go involves differentiating what you can control from what you cannot.

By ceasing to struggle unnecessarily against forces **beyond your control**, you will discover a newfound freedom and become more open to the existing opportunities that you might not see because you are too focused on something else (recall the brown and blue exercise).

This could also be the perfect time to unleash your **creativity** by engaging in artistic activities: writing, music, painting, singing, dancing, etc. Keeping a journal, for example, can help clarify your thoughts and release your emotions.

Humor can also be an excellent way to step back and lighten the circumstances. Don't be afraid to laugh at yourself and the situation. Embrace joy and lightness rather than tension and stiffness. You could, for example, take a few minutes to (re)listen to a comedy sketch that makes you laugh before a meeting you are dreading (which is another form of priming).

Remember that letting go is a personal **skill** that develops over time and with practice. It is up to you to find the techniques and approaches that work best for you. The key is to **persevere** and explore different methods until you find the ones that work best for you on your journey to a more serene state of letting go.

Practicing letting go may take time. Be **patient** with yourself and don't expect instant results. Every small progress counts.

Consider the **support** of a therapist, coach, or support group if you are struggling to let go. They can provide you with personalized tools and guidance.

Letting go will help you find a mental and emotional **balance** while enhancing your overall well-being. By integrating these techniques into your daily life, you will gradually develop a more relaxed, serene, and open attitude towards life and its challenges.

FOR MORE INFORMATION

Atomic Habits: An Easy & Proven Way to Build Good Habits & Break Bad Ones, James Clear, 2018

Awaken the Giant Within: How to Take Immediate Control of Your Mental, Emotional, Physical & Financial Destiny, Anthony Robbins, 1991

Giant Steps: Small Changes to Make a Big Difference, Tony Robbins, 1994

How Should I Start Each Day? What Is Priming? https://www.tonyrobbins.com/ask-tony/priming

Le B.A.-Ba Des Réflexes Archaïques, Emmanuelle Sutherland, 2021

Mind Set Win S2 E1, F1 Champion Max Verstappen On Trusting The Process, https://www.redbull.com/int-en/podcast-episodes/mind-set-win-s2-e1-max-verstappen

Positive Intelligence: Why Only 20% Of Teams And Individuals Achieve Their True Potential And How You Can Achieve Yours, Shirzad Chamine, 2012

Pressing Reset: Original Strength Reloaded, Tim Anderson & Geoff Neupert, 2017

Relations Amoureuses, Familiales ... Se Libérer Des Schémas De Souffrance, avec Franck Lopvet, https://youtu.be/GuoHRy8FBNU?si=MBk9nPeDK38K7nsX

The Big Leap: Conquer Your Hidden Fear and Take Life to The Next Level, Gay Hendricks, 2010

The Body Code: Unlocking Your Body's Ability to Heal Itself, Bradley Nelson, 2023

The Emotion Code: How To Release Your Trapped Emotions for Abundant Health, Love, And Happiness (updated and expanded edition), Bradley Nelson, 2019

The Genius of Athletes: What World-Class Competitors Know That Can Change Your Life, Noel Brick & Scott Douglas, 2021

Unlimited Power, Anthony Robbins, 1986

6 - CONCLUSION

"Life is found in the dance between your deepest desire and your greatest fear."
Tony Robbins

"Changing an organization, a company, a country - or a world - begins with the simple step of changing yourself." Tony Robbins

"Winning is what happens when commitment, desire, talent, preparation, hard work, and leadership all come together." Tom Coughlin

Behind self-mastery and letting go often lies the simple desire to be **happy.**

When **Generation Y** was asked about the most important goal in their lives, over 80% responded "to become rich". And 50% of these same young adults answered "to become famous".

But is that really the most important thing? What if we could analyze entire lives from adolescence to old age to really see what keeps people happy and healthy? Well, that was the goal of a Harvard study on adult development, which is probably the longest study ever conducted on the subject. For 75 years, year after year, researchers followed the lives of 724 men and women, inquiring about their work, family life, and health. In 2015, about 60 of the original 724 participants were still alive, most of them over 90 years old, and still participating in the study. The researchers were even beginning to study their approximately 2,000 children.

THE IMPORTANCE OF RELATIONSHIPS

"There isn't time, so brief is life, for bickerings, apologies, heartburnings, callings to account. There is only time for loving, and but an instant, so to speak, for that." Mark Twain

So, what emerges from the tens of thousands of pages of information collected about these lives? Not wealth, not fame, not even work.

It is, in fact, **good relationships** that make us happier and healthier, while loneliness kills. People who are more socially connected to their families, friends, and communities are happier, healthier, and live longer than those who are less connected.

Above all, the **quality** of your close relationships matters. Conflict-ridden marriages, for example, without much affection, are very bad for our health, perhaps even more so than divorce.

And living in the midst of good, warm relationships seems to protect us from some of the vicissitudes of aging. People who were most satisfied in their relationships at 50 were the healthiest at 80. The happiest couples reported, around 80, that on days when physical pain was strongest, their mood remained just as happy. But for people who were unhappy in their relationships, the days when they reported the most physical pain were exacerbated by more emotional pain.

Good relationships not only protect our bodies, but also protect our **brains**. Being in a securely attached relationship with another person at 80 is protective, and people who are in relationships where they really feel they can rely on the other person if needed have memories that remain sharp for longer. Those in relationships where they do not feel they can count on each other have experienced early declines in memory. Some octogenarian couples could argue continuously, but as long as they knew they could count on each other in tough times, these disputes had no negative effects on their memories.

In his autobiography titled "The Wall", **Vincent Vanasch**, the world's best hockey goalkeeper, also emphasizes the importance of family and friends. Three-time Belgian champion, three-time German champion, double Dutch champion, double club European champion, then European champion, World champion, and Olympic champion with the Red Lions, everything seems to have been simple, beautiful, and great in his career. Yet nothing was a foregone conclusion for the man nicknamed "The Wall", and in his career, there were more defeats than victories. However, he managed to patiently lay each brick of "his wall" on the sole cement of the **family and friends** who supported him at the right moments.

And **you**? What is the quality of your relationships? What if you replaced some screen time with family moments? If you rekindled an old relationship by doing something new together like long walks or evenings, or reached out to that person you haven't spoken to in years, because all these all-too-common quarrels leave a terrible mark on people who hold grudges against each other?

YOUR BIGGEST ENEMY

"Your mind is your best friend, but it is also your worst enemy." *Shirzad Chamine*

According to **Shirzad Chamine**, only 20% of individuals and teams reach their full potential.

Why are New Year's resolutions often forgotten after a few weeks? Why do people who want to lose weight engage in yo-yo diets? Why do we so quickly abandon what we learn in training?

It is because we unconsciously **self-sabotage**. The consequence is not only an impact on the expression of our potential but also a considerable loss of time and energy.

Your mind is **both** your **best friend** and your **worst enemy**. Your success in making the impossible possible will be directly proportional to your ability to tilt the scale in favor of the former.

This can be measured using the **PQ**, the Positive Intelligence Quotient expressed as a percentage from 0 to 100 (calculable for an individual and for a team). This corresponds to the percentage of time during which your mind serves you instead of sabotaging you. A PQ of 75 indicates that your mind serves you 75% of the time and sabotages you during the remaining 25%. This figure of 75 is not insignificant because it represents the tipping point beyond which you must be positioned to be in evolution and not dragged down. You can measure your PQ by visiting the website https://www.positiveintelligence.com.

To improve your PQ, you simply need to learn to **recognize** your saboteurs, **weaken** them, and activate and **strengthen** your "sages", the positive counterparts of the saboteurs. This book is full of principles, strategies, and tools to help you achieve this.

Shirzad Chamine identifies **5 sages** in particular to serve as antidotes:

- the **empathizer** (compassion and understanding towards others and yourself),
- the **explorer** (curiosity and open-mindedness),
- the **innovator** (new perspectives and solutions),
- the **navigator** (the path most aligned with your values and mission), and
- the **activator** (taking action without being disturbed by the saboteurs).

THE LAST WORD

"Why live an ordinary life, when you can live an extraordinary one." Tony Robbins

We have reached the end of this book. I hope that its content has pleased you and that it has allowed you to have a **shift in consciousness** about your ability to achieve your wildest dreams.

Remember that self-mastery and letting go are two sides of the same coin and complement each other perfectly depending on the circumstances.

See **self-mastery** as increasing your own standards and **letting go** as decreasing your expectations of others and external circumstances.

Lastly, keep in mind that making the impossible possible is an **endless and limitless path**, which is what makes it so beautiful, and that your success will depend on your ability to make it a lifestyle.

If you enjoyed this book, please leave a positive review on Amazon. It would greatly help its distribution. Thank you in advance!

*"Let me tell you something you already know. The world ain't all sunshine and rainbows, it's a very mean and nasty place and I don't care how tough you are, it will beat you to your knees and keep you there permanently if you let it. You, me or nobody is going to hit as hard as life but it ain't about how hard you hit, it's about how hard you can get hit and keep moving forward, how much you can take and keep moving forward. That's how winning is done. Now if you know what you're worth to, go out and get what you're worth but you gotta be willing to take the hits and not pointing fingers saying you ain't where you want to be because of him or her or anybody. Cowards do that and that ain't you, **you're better than that**."* - Rocky Balboa, 2006

FOR MORE INFORMATION

Positive Intelligence: Why Only 20% Of Teams And Individuals Achieve Their True Potential And How You Can Achieve Yours, Shirzad Chamine, 2012

Rocky Balboa, 2006, https://www.youtube.com/watch?v=D_Vg4uyYwEk

The Big Leap: Conquer Your Hidden Fear and Take Life to The Next Level, Gay Hendricks, 2010

The Wall, Vincent Vanasch, 2023

What Makes a Good Life? Lessons From The Longest Study On Happiness, Robert Waldinger, TEDxBeaconStreet, 2015, https://www.ted.com/talks/robert_waldinger_what_makes_a_good_life_lessons_from_the_longest_study_on_happiness/transcript

7 - ABOUT THE AUTHOR

I like to say that I lived two parallel lives until 2017, when I started to combine the two.

After a master's degree in biochemistry followed by a doctorate, I worked for about twenty years in various Research & Development environments (university, SMEs, a multinational company & a hospital reference center).

A life at 200 miles per hour where I notably learned team and project management as well as strategic outsourcing (with all that implies in terms of governance, performance management, risks and issues management, quality, legal aspects, and procurement). I also experienced toxic management, biased evaluations, and abusive layoffs. All of this gave me a deep desire to learn how to manage differently and become a recognized agent of change in the field.

Karate (of which I am currently a 4th degree black belt) and functional training (mainly at home) allowed me to stay on course during the more difficult times. I also had the opportunity to practice aikido, qi gong, yoga, and CrossFit. Over the years, I have observed individual and collective performance issues and have trained in communication in the broadest sense. It was a real revelation, and I realized that it was what truly motivated me.

In 2017, at the age of 44, a trip to the south of France and a CrossFit training inspired me to take action and train with the world's best. I then followed and obtained several coaching certifications in different areas to better understand and thus express all my potential.

I also discovered Biohacking, of which I have become a big fan, and which, in a way, connects my two lives. By combining ancestral knowledge (especially martial arts) and the most advanced scientific disciplines, it allows us to function optimally by providing many solutions to our modern daily constraints.

In 2021, I experienced difficult moments both personally and professionally. I then deepened the notions of resilience and antifragility, respectively through the work of **Boris Cyrulnik** and **Nassim Nicholas Taleb**. Today, richer and stronger from all these experiences, I support individuals and organizations who want to regain control and improve their results in both their personal and professional lives.

Laurent Zecchinon

Website

https://laurentzecchinon.com

Facebook Page (in French)

https://www.facebook.com/lzecchinon.coaching.biohacking

YouTube Channel (in French)

Laurent Zecchinon - Coaching & Biohacking
https://www.youtube.com/channel/UCFZc-S7wxQgUMG_EufSIz6w

Linkedin Profile

https://www.linkedin.com/in/laurent-zecchinon/

8 - REFERENCES

1. Abraham Lincoln,
   https://en.wikipedia.org/wiki/Abraham_Lincoln

2. Antifragile: Things That Gain from Disorder, Nassim Nicholas Taleb, 2014

3. Atomic Habits: An Easy & Proven Way to Build Good Habits & Break Bad Ones, James Clear, 2018

4. Awaken the Giant Within: How to Take Immediate Control of Your Mental, Emotional, Physical & Financial Destiny, Anthony Robbins, 1991

5. Boundless: Upgrade Your Brain, Optimize Your Body & Defy Aging, Ben Greenfield, 2020

6. Depression, Daily Stressors And Inflammatory Responses To High-Fat Meals : When Stress Overrides Healthier Food Choices. Kiecolt-Glaser et al, Molecular Psychiatry (2017) 22, 476-482
   (https://nature.com/articles/mp2016149.epdf)

7. Earthing - Connexion à la Terre - Live avec Hugues Ostoja-Kuczynski,
   https://youtube.com/live/8k7ZSoVnyBM?feature=share

8. Et Si Votre Maison Troublait Votre Sommeil ? Hugues Ostoja-Kuczynski, 2020

9. Experiencing Physical Warmth Promotes Interpersonal Warmth, Lawrence E. Williams And John A. Bargh, Science, Vol 322 (24 Oct 2008), Issue 5901: 606-607

10. Four Powerful Mindsets of Karate, Jesse Enkamp,
    https://youtu.be/QjZ3IhHqBY8?si=1D_f3eS4d6qXs_bM

11. Giant Steps: Small Changes to Make A Big Difference, Tony Robbins, 1994

12. Hanuman's Figurine Is President Barack Obama's Lucky Charm, 2016, https://economictimes.indiatimes.com/news/politics-and-nation/hanuman-figurine-is-president-barack-obamas-lucky-charm/articleshow/50603496.cms

13. How Should I Start Each Day? What Is Priming? https://www.tonyrobbins.com/ask-tony/priming

14. Le B.A.-Ba Des Réflexes Archaïques, Emmanuelle Sutherland, 2021

15. L'effet Placebo En Toute Transparence, Kheira Bettayeb, 2023, https://lejournal.cnrs.fr/articles/leffet-placebo-en-toute-transparence

16. Les Vertus De L'échec, Charles Pépin, 2018

17. Life Force: How New Breakthroughs In Precision Medicine Can Transform The Quality Of Your Life & Those You Love, Tony Robbins, 2022

18. Man's Search for Meaning: The Classic Tribute to Hope from The Holocaust, Viktor Frankl, 2004

19. Mind Map Mastery: The Complete Guide to Learning and Using the Most Powerful Thinking Tool in The Universe, Tony Buzan, 2018

20. Mindset: The New Psychology of Success, Carol S. Dweck, 2007

21. Mind Set Win S2 E1, F1 Champion Max Verstappen On

Trusting The Process, https://www.redbull.com/int-en/podcast-episodes/mind-set-win-s2-e1-max-verstappen

22. Modeling with NLP, Robert Dilts, 1998

23. Neurotransmetteurs et Nutrition du Stress, https://www.pensersante.fr/neurotransmetteurs-nutrition-du-stress

24. On The Malignant Transformation Of Cells During Prolonged Culture Under Hypoxic Conditions *in vitro,* Harry Goldblatt, Libby Friedman, Ronald L. Cechner, Biochemical Medicine, Volume 7, Issue 2, April 1973, Pages 241-252, https://www.sciencedirect.com/science/article/abs/pii/0006294473900793

25. Peak: How All of Us Can Achieve Extraordinary Things, Anders Ericsson & Robert Pool, 2017

26. Positive Intelligence: Why Only 20% Of Teams And Individuals Achieve Their True Potential And How You Can Achieve Yours, Shirzad Chamine, 2012

27. Power Posing Is Back: Amy Cuddy Successfully Refutes Criticism, Kim Elsesser, 2018, https://www.forbes.com/sites/kimelsesser/2018/04/03/power-posing-is-back-amy-cuddy-successfully-refutes-criticism/?sh=686dd79d3b8e

28. Pressing Reset: Original Strength Reloaded, Tim Anderson & Geoff Neupert, 2017

29. Relations Amoureuses, Familiales ... Se Libérer Des Schémas De Souffrance, avec Franck Lopvet,

https://youtu.be/GuoHRy8FBNU?si=MBk9nPeDK38K7nsX

30. Rocky Balboa, 2006,
https://www.youtube.com/watch?v=D_Vg4uyYwEk

31. Self-Discipline: The Spartan and Special Operations Way to Mastering Yourself, Ryan Hunt, 2019

32. Siri Lindley, https://en.wikipedia.org/wiki/Siri_Lindley

33. Success Factor Modeling Volumes I-III, Robert Brian Dilts and Antonio Meza, 2015-2017

34. The Big Leap: Conquer Your Hidden Fear and Take Life to The Next Level, Gay Hendricks, 2010

35. The Body Code: Unlocking Your Body's Ability to Heal Itself, Bradley Nelson, 2023

36. The Code of the Extraordinary Mind: 10 Unconventional Laws to Redefine Your Life and Succeed on Your Own Terms, Vishen Lakhiani, 2016

37. The Emotion Code: How to Release Your Trapped Emotions for Abundant Health, Love, and Happiness (Updated and Expanded Edition), Bradley Nelson, 2019

38. The Functional Medicine Tree, Frank Lipman,
https://youtu.be/DBdFq9O3W-8?si=_YrlMJgcwZlSmHuf

39. The Genius of Athletes: What World-Class Competitors Know That Can Change Your Life, Noel Brick & Scott Douglas, 2021

40. The Law of Polarity, Tony Robbins,
https://www.tonyrobbins.com/ask-tony/polarity/

41. The Power of Full Engagement, Jim Loehr & Tony Schwartz, 2003

42. The Power of Mindset Change: Why Mindset Matters Most, Robert B Dilts & Mickey Feher, 2023

43. The Power of When: Discover Your Chronotype--and the Best Time to Eat Lunch, Ask for a Raise, Have Sex, Write a Novel, Take Your Meds, and More, Michael Breus, 2016

44. The Seeker's Code: Your Access to The Unreasonable and Extraordinary, Donny Epstein, 2023

45. The Wall, Vincent Vanasch, 2023

46. To Me, To You: How You Say Things Matters for Endurance Performance, James Hardy, Aled V. Thomas, and Anthony W. Blanchfield, Journal of Sports Sciences 37, no 18 (September 2019): 2122-30

47. Tout sur les Chakras ou Presque, Céline Miconnet, 2019, https://blog.green-yoga.fr/tout-sur-chakras-ou-presque/

48. Unlimited Power, Anthony Robbins, 1986

49. Un Optimiste Persévérant : Abraham Lincoln, https://www.liguedesoptimistes.fr/2012/10/28/un-optimiste-perseverant-abraham-lincoln

50. Voluntary Activation of The Sympathetic Nervous System and Attenuation of The Innate Immune Response in Humans. Kox et al, Proceedings of the National Academy of Sciences USA (2014) 111 (20) 7379-84 (https://ncbi.nlm.nih.gov/pubmed/24799686)

51. What Makes a Good Life? Lessons From The Longest

Study On Happiness, Robert Waldinger, TEDxBeaconStreet, 2015, https://www.ted.com/talks/robert_waldinger_what_makes_a_good_life_lessons_from_the_longest_study_on_happiness/transcript

52. Why We Do What We Do, Tony Robbins, 2006, TED talk, https://www.ted.com/talks/tony_robbins_why_we_do_what_we_do

53. Wim Hof Method, https://www.wimhofmethod.com

54. Woman Code: Perfect Your Cycle, Amplify Your Fertility, Supercharge Your Sex Drive and Become a Power Source, Alisa Vitti, 2013

55. Your Body Language May Shape Who You Are, Amy Cuddy, 2012, TED talk, https://www.ted.com/talks/amy_cuddy_your_body_languag-may_shape_who_you_are/transcript